THE ENERGY SOLUTION:

Nutrients to fire up your energy metabolism for sustained energy release

Copyright © Jan Clementson 2015

Author: Jan Clementson
BSc (Hons) Nut Med
mBANT, CNHC registered
https://www.facebook.com/TheEnergySolutionEbook

Cover Designer: Kerman Rodriguez
www.coversdesigner.com

Disclaimer

All rights reserved. No part of this book may be reproduced in any form or by any electronic or mechanical means including information storage and retrieval systems – except in the case of brief quotations embodied in critical articles or reviews – without the permission in writing from its publisher. This publication is designed to provide accurate and authorative information in regard to the subject matter covered, with the understanding that the publisher is not engaged in rendering legal, accounting or other professional service.

This book is not intended as a substitute for medical guidance from a qualified doctor/healthcare practitioner. The intent of this book is to offer accurate general information in regard to the subject matter covered. If medical advice or other expert help is required, the services of a proper medical professional should be sought. If you are on any medications, seek advice from a medical practitioner before consuming any nutritional supplements as possible interactions can occur that can affect the effectiveness of the medication.

Table of Contents

Preface 6

PART ONE: The Science 7

Chapter 1: Introduction 8

Chapter 2: Energy 10
    What is Energy? 10
    Energy Metabolism 11
    Energy Homeostasis 11
    Energy Sources 12
    Energy Production 15
    Cellular Respiration 16
    Energy Disruption 17

Chapter 3: Symptoms 18
    Fatigue 18
    Dehydration 19
    Blood Sugar Instability 20
    Categories of Blood Sugar Instability 21
    Stress 23
    General Adaptation Syndrome 25
    Chronic Fatigue Syndrome (CFS) 27

Chapter 4: Medical Management 29
    Fatigue 29
    Dehydration 30
    Blood Sugar Instability 30
    Stress 31
    Chronic Fatigue Syndrome 31

Chapter 5: Pathophysiology 33
    Energy Demand 33
    Cellular Energy Production 33
    Cellular Respiration 34

Circadian Regulation 35

Nervous System Regulation 37

Hormone Regulation 38

Brain Regulatory Control 41

Chapter 6: Clinical Considerations 42

Where to Start? 42

Stress 42

Blood Sugar Control 43

The Gastrointestinal (GI) Tract 43

Adrenal Over-Stimulation 45

Inflammation 46

Thyroid Imbalance 47

Mitochondrial Dysfunction 48

Environmental Toxic Exposure 49

PART TWO: The Energy Programme Plan 51

Overview 51

Chapter 7: Hydration 52

The Starting Point 52

Water Requirements 52

The Electrolytes 52

Quick Reference Dehydration Chart 54

Key Action Points 55

Chapter 8: Sleep 56

Sleep Deprivation 56

Biological Function 56

The Sleep-Wake Cycle 57

Jetlag and Shift Work 58

Sleep Hygiene 58

General Sleeping Tips 59

Chapter 9: Stress Management 63

Stress Response 63

Stress Source Identification 64

Stress Journal 64

Stress Coping Methods 64

Change Instigation 65

Stress Management Strategies 65

Chapter 10: Diet 68

The Goal 68

Set Yourself up for Success 69

Carbohydrates 70

Fats 72

Proteins 74

Sugar Overload 76

Food Timing 77

Key Action Points 78

Chapter 11: The Case for Supplements 79

Hype or Help? 79

The Food Chain Supply 79

Environmental Toxin Exposure 80

Age, Exercise and Stress 81

Misleading News Stories 81

The Scientific Evidence 82

Statistics 83

The Supplement Market 84

Natural vs Synthetic Supplements 85

Supplement Brands 86

Chapter 12: Specific Supplements 87

Health Foundation Supplements 87

    The Basics 87

    Multi-Vitamins and Minerals 87

    Probiotics 89

    Milk Thistle (AKA Silymarin) 90

    Vitamin C (AKA Ascorbic Acid) 92

Energy Specific Supplements 93

    Cellular Energy Nutrients 93

    Magnesium and Calcium 94

    B Vitamins 95

    Alpha-Lipoic Acid, L-Carnitine and CoQ10 97

    Creatine 100

    Omega-3 Fats 102

  Summary 103

Chapter 13: Exercise 105

  Health Consequences of Inactivity 105

  The Energy Systems 105

  Energy Fuel 106

  Blood Glucose Maintenance 107

  Exercise and Fatigue 108

  Stress and Adrenal Fatigue 109

  Exercise Recommendations 110

Chapter 14: Stimulants 112

  Caffeine 112

  Energy Drinks 114

  Alcohol 115

  Key Points 119

Chapter 15: Conclusion 120

  Overview 120

  Energy Definitions 120

  Energy Dynamics 121

  Energy Disruption 122

  The Energy Programme Plan in a Nutshell 125

  Final Thought 127

About the Author 128

  Jan Clementson 128

References 129

Preface

The background to this book started many years ago in my childhood. Having suffered from 'growing pains' as a child, I eventually discovered that it was an intolerance to dairy, and cheese in particular, that was causing the problems. There began my understanding of the connection between food and health. This was further strengthened by my years as a competitive athlete for my local running club where I started to notice how my energy levels and performance changed with different foods. Fast forward a few years and I began working for a book publishing company (The Random House Group) in the health and fitness division. Here, I was inspired to follow my true passion for nutrition and health and returned to university to study Nutritional Medicine, where I obtained a first-class honours degree. After graduation, I worked as a Clinical Nutrition Advisor for a professional nutritional supplement company (BioCare Ltd).

It was at BioCare that I was able to develop my interest in biochemical mechanisms and energy dynamics in particular. As my understanding of these mechanisms grew, I started to explain them to customers when advising on specific health conditions. The overwhelming positive responses were staggering. People were so delighted to have an explanation for what was happening in their bodies and why, that they were incentivised to follow my advice. It was clear to me that people wanted to take charge of their own health. The trend was so noticeable that I aspired to reach a wider audience who could benefit from my understanding and knowledge. And so this is the basis of how this book came into being.

With this book, I am to inspire and encourage you to take charge of your own health and improve the quality of your life so that you can be the best that you can be. I have set up a Facebook page for followers of this book and would dearly love to hear your comments, including how this book has impacted on the quality of your life. The Facebook page is: https://www.facebook.com/TheEnergySolutionEbook.

Acknowledgements

With sincere thanks to my family and friends who supported me during this process and through a time of transition.

PART ONE:
The Science

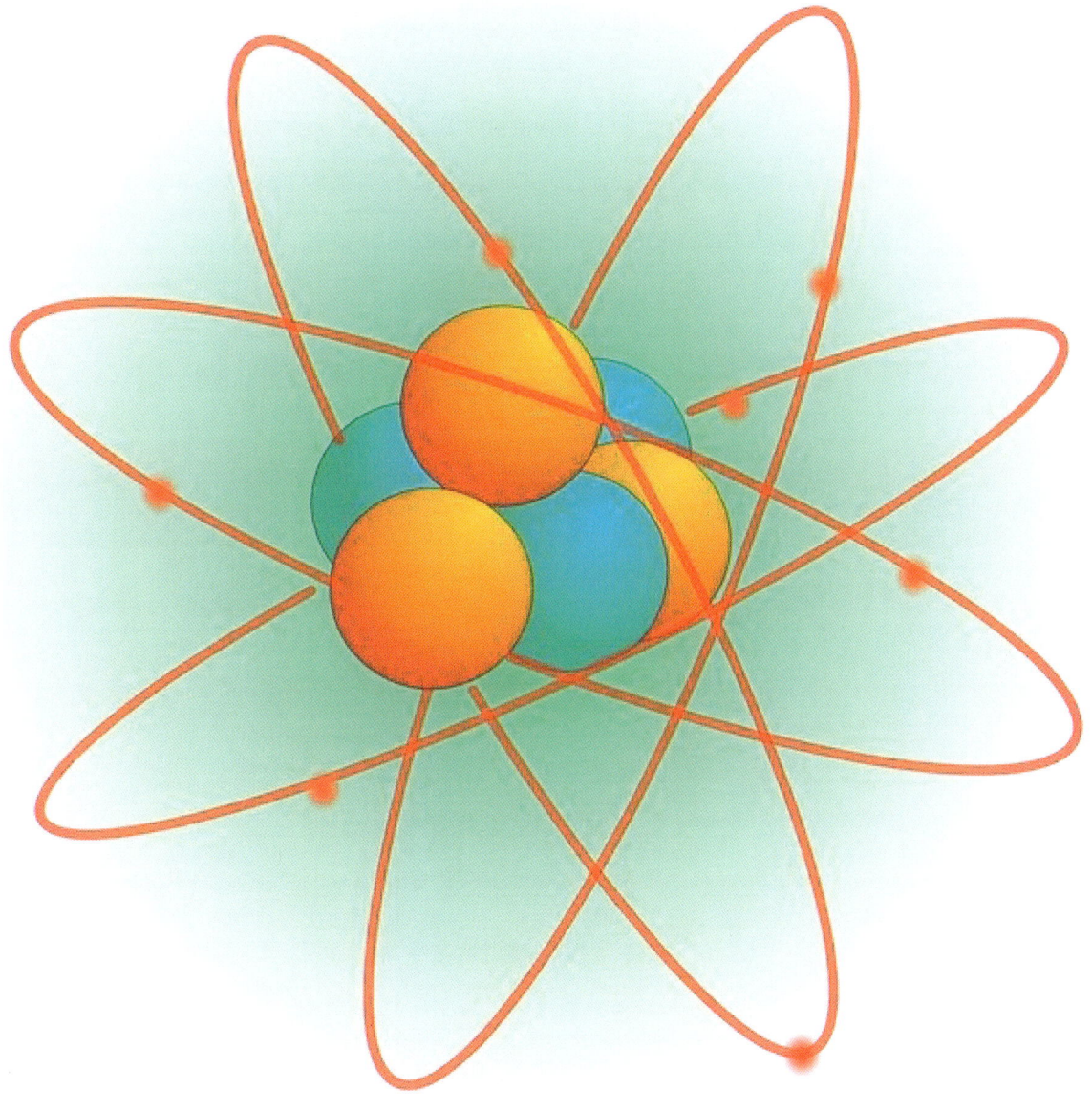

Source: www.pixabay.com

Chapter 1: Introduction

Fatigue is becoming an energy-draining epidemic that underlies a growing human energy crisis. Today's society has become a multi-tasking, over-scheduled culture with very few boundaries between our personal and professional lives. Increased workload, stress, junk food, inactivity, and sleep deprivation are all impacting our energy levels. Coinciding with this change in culture is the growing rise of energy related disorders from obesity (excess energy storage) to the **metabolic syndrome** (a disorder of energy utilisation and storage). The latter encompasses abdominal obesity; and elevated blood pressure, blood sugar and blood fats; with increased risk of diabetes and cardiovascular disease. All of which are now prevalent in Western society.

What is becoming very clear is the need to understand the physiological basis of metabolism to tackle the energy drain. In the past, the idea of achieving energy balance was thought of in simplistic terms as the energy intake versus the energy expenditure:

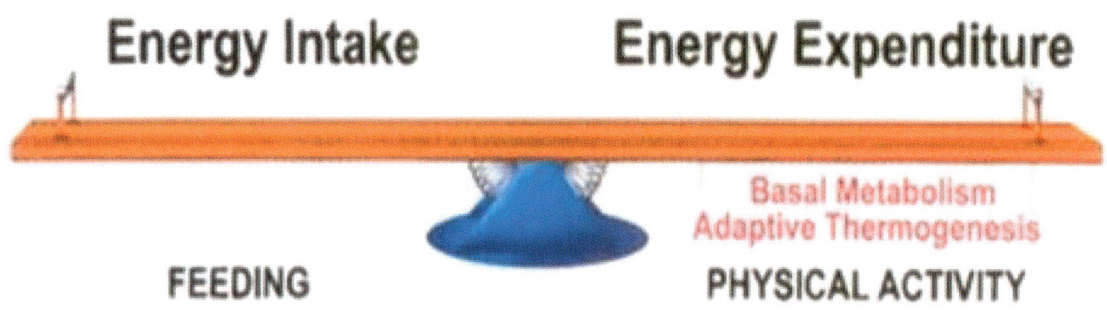

Source: Cell (2001) 104(4): 531-543[1]

To a certain extent, this is correct but it is too simplistic. Feeding behaviour lies at the interface between free will and physiology but it is influenced by many factors including food availability and composition; metabolic, neural and endocrine factors; and is modified by powerful visual, olfactory, emotional and cognitive inputs.[2] It is now widely recognised that energy storage results from an interaction between genetic, environmental and psychosocial factors. It is these influences that ultimately change the energy balance equation via a brain-controlled homeostatic regulatory mechanism.

Advances in the scientific understanding of the metabolic regulatory pathways over the past decade are now starting to provide a roadmap to better address energy balance on an individual level. This book seeks to educate and raise awareness of the dynamics of energy balance, whilst providing a practical programme plan that will help you to integrate the science into your own lives to achieve optimal energy levels.

Chapter 2: Energy

What is Energy?

We all know the term "energy" and we all know how it feels to have energy or to be lacking in energy. But do you actually know what energy is? In the terms of physics, it can be described as ***the property of an object which can be converted from one form to another but cannot be created or destroyed***.[3] The energy itself already exists; it is simply transformed or transferred from one state to another through physical interactions.

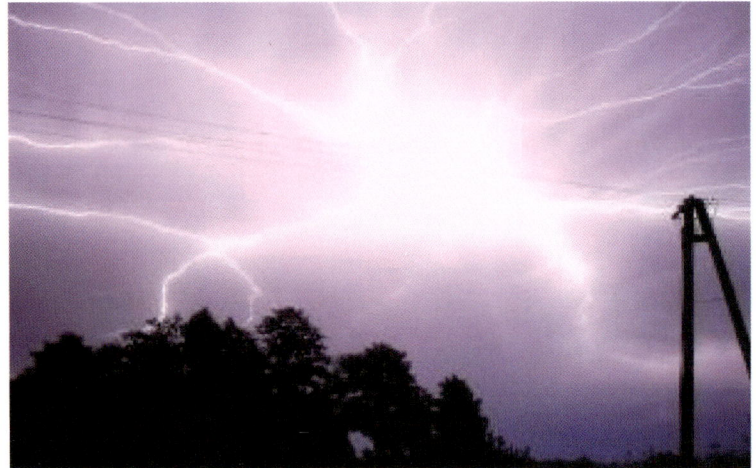
Source: www.freeimages.com

This potential energy exists in many forms, such as the **kinetic** energy of a moving object, the **radiant** energy carried by light or the **thermal** energy carried by heat. Typical lightning strikes can covert 500 MJ of electrical energy into other forms of energy, such as light, sound and heat. It is this **'potential energy'** that enables the world to function and survive – radiant energy from the sun and geothermal energy from the earth drives our climate and ecosystem; food energy sustains life for humans and organisms; whilst fossil fuel energy powers our civilisation.

Ultimately, we receive our energy from the environment. Plants take in nutrients directly from the soil through their roots and from the atmosphere through their leaves. When we eat these plants we break down their structures through our specialised digestive systems that releases energy stored within. Our bodies then use that energy to transform it into biological energy; which is responsible for our growth, development, functioning, reproduction and life itself. Without energy, we would cease to exist.

Energy Metabolism

Biological energy production occurs through a set of chemical reactions within our cells called *metabolism*. These chemical reactions are organized into metabolic pathways, in which one chemical is transformed through a series of steps into another chemical by a sequence of enzymes. These enzymes are crucial because they are the catalysts that drive the reactions. Metabolism is usually divided into two categories: *catabolism*, which breaks down matter to release energy; and *anabolism*, which uses energy to construct matter. The purpose of a catabolic reaction is to provide the energy and components needed by anabolic reactions. Hence, energy production is a catabolic process.

Catabolsim	• Breaks down matter to release energy
Anabolism	• Uses energy to construct matter

The metabolic system determines which substances will be nutritious and which poisonous. The speed of metabolism is called the *metabolic rate* and it is this rate that influences how much food you will require and how quickly you will burn off the food as energy. Metabolic reactions focus on the **macronutrients** *(carbohydrates, fats and proteins)* by either breaking them down and using them as a source of energy or using their basic components to build cells and tissues.

Energy Homeostasis

For you to function properly, your energy needs to be kept in balance. Your body does this through a process called *energy homeostasis.* This balances your energy intake with your energy output, energy storage, work that you do, and heat that you release. It can be measured with the following equation:[4]

Energy Intake = Energy Output = Energy Stored + Work + Heat

This biological energy is expressed using the energy unit *calorie (cal),* which relates to the *energy needed to increase the temperature of 1 kg of water by 1°C.*[5] Most of us have all heard of the calorie, many of us even count the calories in food to maintain or lose weight; and whether you realise it or not, you are aware that some sort of energy transfer happens when you eat food. So when you eat a calorie of food, it is either: (1) stored as fat (hence the associations with weight gain); (2) transferred to the body's cellular batteries for energy production for mechanical work or chemical synthesis; or (3) dissipated as heat.

Metabolic Pathways of Food Energy
1. Stored as fat; or
2. Transferred to your cellular energy batteries for energy production; or
3. Dissipated as heat

The amount of energy flowing into each of these three pathways is controlled by hormonal and neuronal signals; which in turn, regulate calorie intake through the sensations of hunger and satiety.[6] Hence, food intake, energy expenditure and body fat are internally regulated to ensure that your bodily systems remain stable and relatively constant.[7]

Energy Sources

Carbohydrates are the major fuel source for metabolism. They are made up of types of sugars that can be divided into **simple** and **complex** carbohydrates. Simple sugars consist of single or double sugar units called *monosaccharides* (such as glucose and fructose) and *disaccharides* (such as sucrose and lactose); whereas complex carbohydrates consist of three or more sugar units linked in a chain and are termed *oligosaccharides* and *polysaccharides* (such as starch, glycogen, and cellulose). Metabolising **one gram of carbohydrate** yields approximately **4 kcal of energy**.

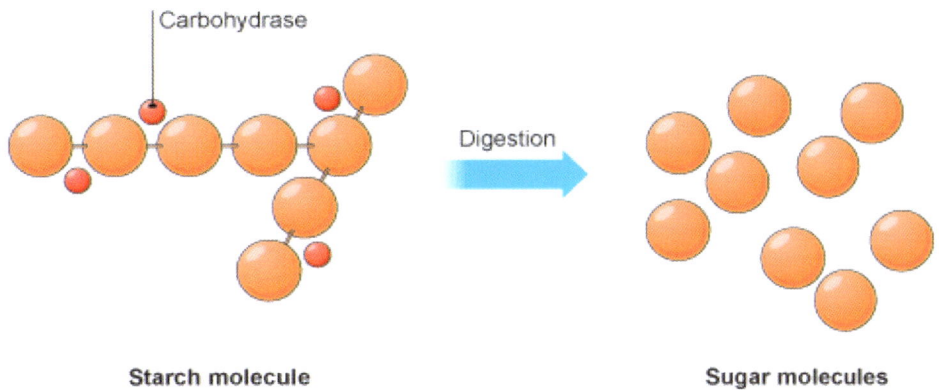

Starch molecule → Sugar molecules

Source: www.bbc.co.uk/bitesize

All carbohydrates will break down in your body to a single **sugar unit** *(monosaccharide)*, of which there are three: *glucose, fructose* and *galactose*. However, it is **glucose** that is the main sugar unit and also the metabolic regulator. It is the concentration of glucose in the blood that acts as the main control for the metabolic hormone **insulin**, which directs glucose to the cells to either be used for energy or towards storage. Storage is firstly as **glycogen** in the liver and muscles to act as a readily available energy source, and then as *fat* for longer-term storage.

Fats are a subgroup of lipids called triglycerides and are the main storage form of energy.[8] They can hold more than six times the amount of energy per storage mass than carbohydrates because they are stored in a relatively water-free environment - unlike carbohydrates which are more hydrated. This allows for a greater energy yield when metabolised, equating to approximately **9 kcal per gram**.[9] The fat cells in which they are held are designed for continuous synthesis and breakdown of triglycerides, with their breakdown being controlled by the hormone sensitive enzyme **lipase**.[10]

Triglycerides consist of three **fatty acids** (basic fat units) – chains of hydrogen and carbon molecules - attached to a sugar molecule (glycerol). When these chains contain one or more double bonds between the carbon and hydrogen molecules, the fatty acids are called **unsaturated fats**; when only single bonds occur, the fatty acids are termed **saturated fats**. Saturated fats are found in animal fats, processed meats, butter, cheese and coconut oil; whereas unsaturated fats are found in oily fish, nuts, seeds and olive oil.

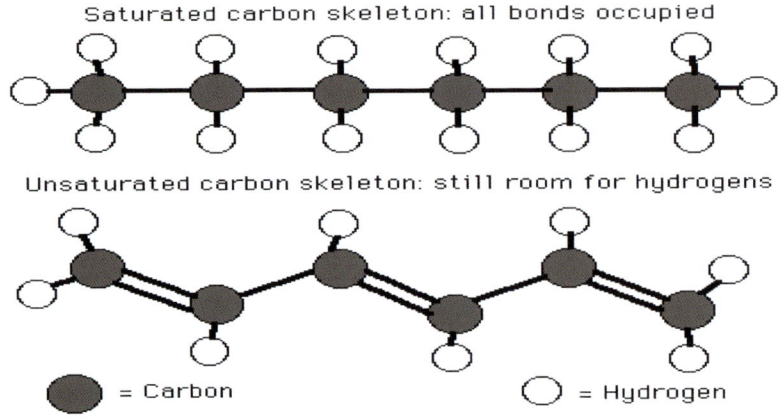

Source: www.staff.jccc.net

Fatty acids from foods are usually ingested as triglycerides. Because these cannot be absorbed by the intestine,[11] they are broken down in the digestive system (by bile and the pancreatic enzyme lipase) into free fatty acids and glycerol, which can be used in metabolism. However, because fatty acids cannot be converted to glucose (the main fuel of the body), they are metabolised via a different pathway within the cell to yield energy.[12]

Proteins are long chains of ***amino acids*** (basic building blocks) that perform a vast array of functions. They differ from one another primarily in their sequence of amino acids. Through the process of digestion, proteins are broken down into free amino acids that are then used in metabolism. Their best known role in the cell is as enzymes, which catalyse chemical reactions. Over 4,000 reactions are known to be catalysed by enzymes,[13] whilst almost all of the reactions involved in metabolism are enzyme-induced. The rate acceleration conferred by enzymatic catalysis is often enormous - as much as 10^{17}-fold increase.[14] Hence, they are vital to metabolism.

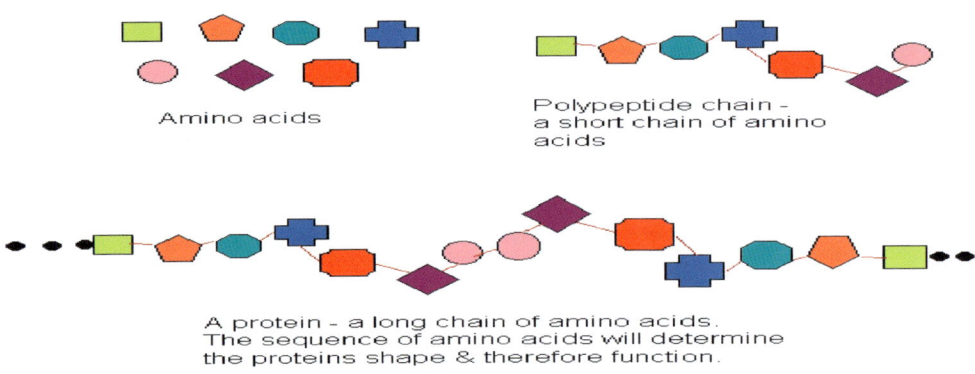

Source: www.lenahealth.blogspot.com

There are twenty standard amino acids, some of which are termed "essential" because they cannot be synthesised in the body and so must come from the diet.[15] Some of these amino acids can be converted to glucose through a process called *gluconeogenesis*, which allows them to be used as a fuel source where they yield approximately **4 kcal of energy per gram**. This use of protein as a fuel is particularly important under starvation conditions as it allows the body's own proteins to be used to support life, particularly those found in muscle.[16] However, proteins are the least favourite fuel to use for energy production because of their importance in enzyme synthesis and cell and organ structure, in addition to them being harder to break down because of their more complex structure.

Fuel Source Priority

Your body will use the available fuel sources in the following order of priority:

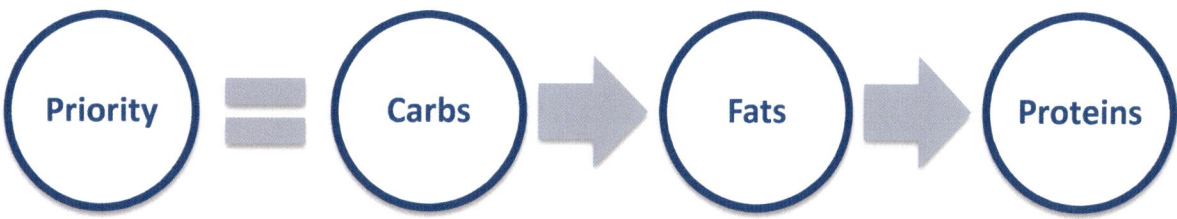

Energy Production

It is the function of *metabolism* (chemical transformations within cells) that enables you to transfer the potential energy from your fuel sources into biological energy that will power your body. The process begins with digestion where your specialised digestive system breaks down foods into their constituent parts - carbohydrates are broken down to glucose; fats are broken down to fatty acids; and proteins are broken down to amino acids. These constituent parts are then absorbed into the blood from the small intestine.

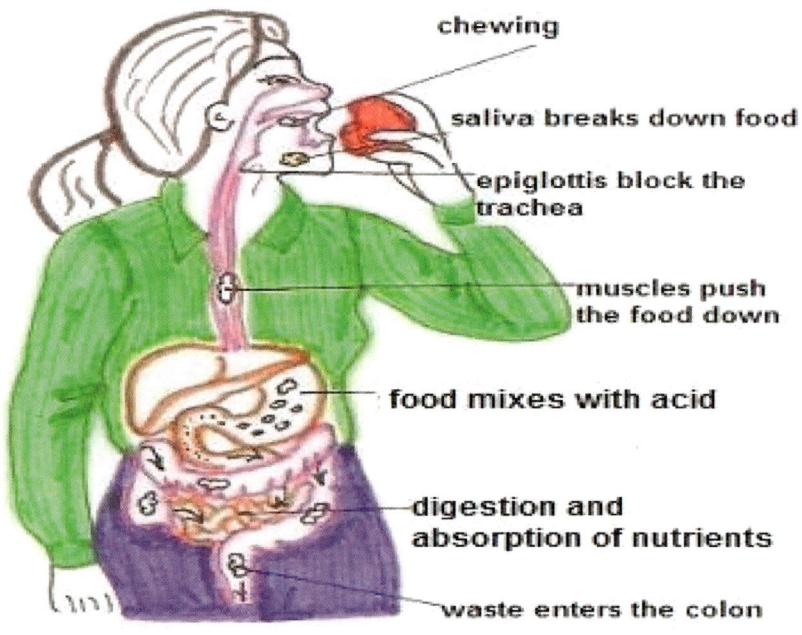

Source: www.health-lesson-plans-teacher.com

Once the food components are in the blood stream they can then be carried around the body to be utilised by the cells for energy production. It is inside the cells themselves that energy is transferred or 'produced' in a process called *cellular respiration.*[17] This process stores energy temporarily within the cells in the form of **ATP (adenosine triphosphate)**, which is the **energy currency of the body.**[18]

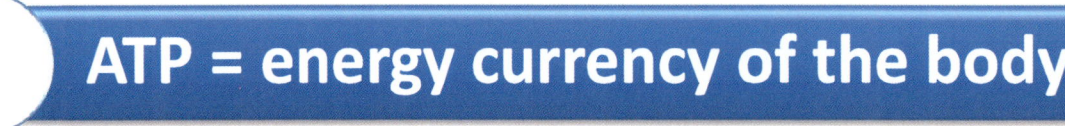

Cellular Respiration

The energy transfer from food occurs inside your cells through multiple enzymatic reactions occurring in a set sequence, which produce electrical energy that can be converted into biological energy. Glucose, fatty acids and amino acids are converted into an intermediary molecule called *acetyl-CoA,* which feeds directly into a two-step process – firstly the **Citric Acid**

Cycle (AKA Krebs Cycle) and then the *Electron Transport Chain* - to produce energy in the form of ATP. **It is ATP that is the energy carrier or energy currency** of the body and transports chemical energy within cells.[19] The overall process can produce about 30 molecules of ATP from a single molecule of glucose.[20] However, each ATP molecule needs to be continuously recycled - at the rate of about 500 to 750 times per day[21] - because the molecule cannot store energy long-term.

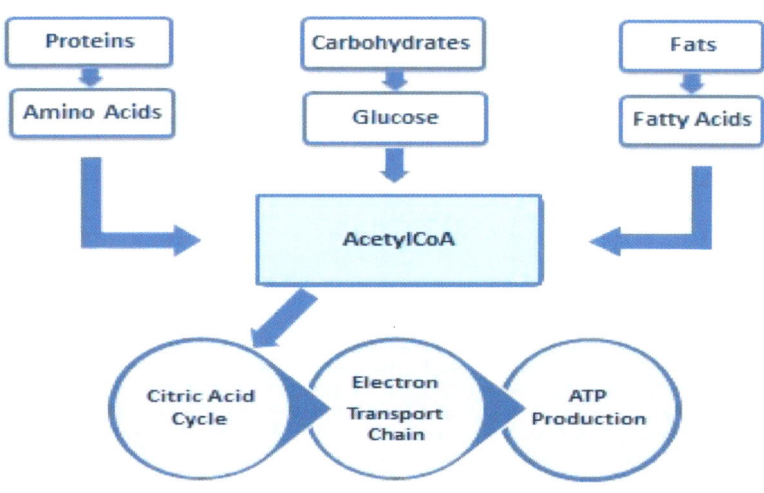

Energy Production Mechanism

Energy Disruption

This highly complex process of energy transfer involves a symphony of inter-linked nutritional, chemical, hormonal and neurotransmitter (nerve) messages that provide and modulate fuel delivery and utilisation. These inter-linking systems can all be disrupted for a variety of reasons. So, although energy cannot be destroyed, the actual process of energy transfer, or 'energy production', can be disrupted; which can lead to disturbed energy conditions that are endemic within society today. This book seeks to guide you through the myriad possible scenarios that can lead to such energy disruption, whilst showing you how to re-balance your systems and prevent negative energy balance.

Chapter 3: Symptoms

Fatigue

Fatigue is a term that is readily used these days to describe tiredness or a lack of energy. It is essentially a general name that can include exhaustion, tiredness and listlessness; and is very much a subjective feeling, which has a gradual onset. ***Fatigue symptoms are broadly found on three levels: physical, mental and emotional.*** Physical effects include yawning, eye rubbing, slumped posture and an increased likelihood of falling asleep. Mental effects manifest as slow responses; so you take longer to do mental work and are more likely to make mistakes. Emotionally, you are likely to become grumpy, unaffectionate, irritable, short-tempered, terse and uncommunicative.

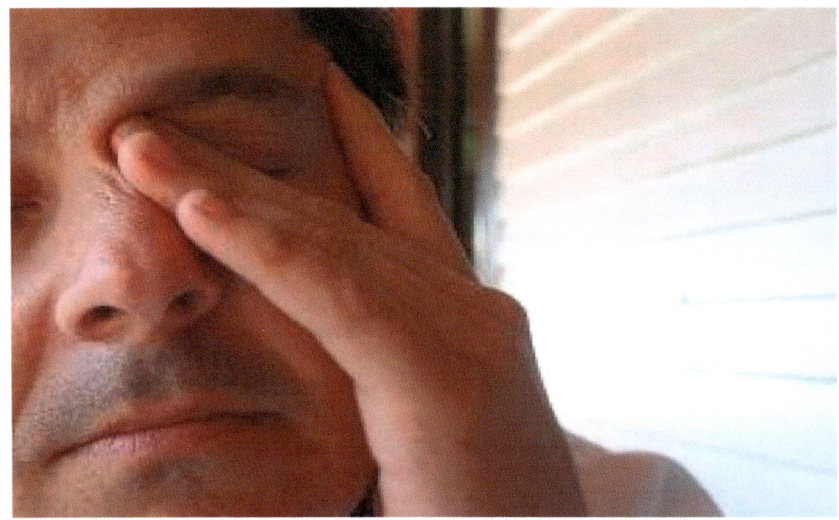

Source: www.freeimages.com

Often, such feelings can be alleviated by periods of rest, although it is becoming increasingly common in today's society for such feelings to persist despite sufficient rest. Medically, fatigue is treated as a non-specific symptom, which means that it has many possible causes. As such, it is the worst treated symptom of conventional medicine. The level of fatigue can range from mild tiredness to *Chronic Fatigue Syndrome (CFS)*, which is a particularly severe form of fatigue. However, no matter what your level of fatigue, you can improve your energy levels, performance and efficiency.

Dehydration

Dehydration is much overlooked when addressing fatigue symptoms, yet it is a common factor that can easily result in tiredness or a lack of energy. It occurs when water loss exceeds water intake. Most people can tolerate a 3-4% decrease in body water, although symptoms generally become noticeable after a 2% decrease.[22] At a decrease of only 1%, there will be a measurable effect on body temperature regulation in response to exercise; a 2-3% reduction will impair exercise performance; whilst a 6-7% reduction can cause fatigue and dizziness, and lead to a life-threatening situation.[23] More than a 15% decrease is invariably fatal as organs start to fail.[24]

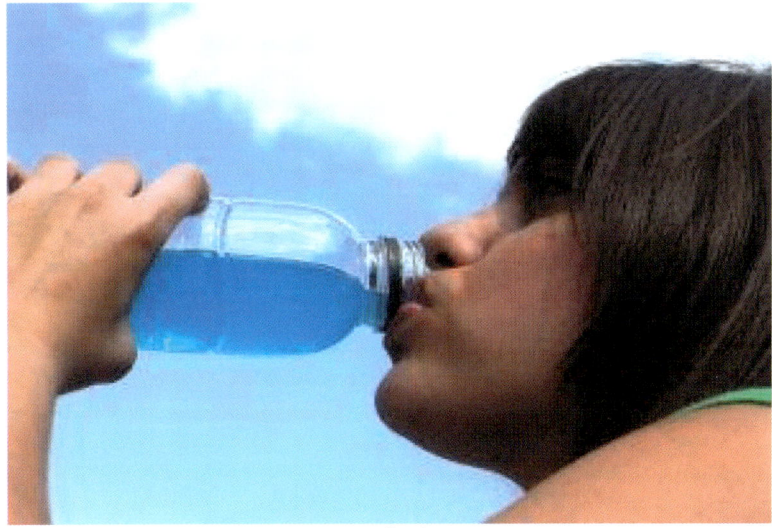

Source: www.freeimages.com

Water can have such a major impact on energy levels because it performs multiple functions. It is critical to all metabolic processes; carries nutrients and wastes around the body; acts as a solvent for the dissolution of molecules; lubricates joints, the spine and the brain; and regulates temperature through sweating. Plus, regular water consumption is necessary to replace the water lost through urine, faeces, sweating and the breath. And with physical exertion and heat exposure, water loss will increase.

Dehydration → Body temp jumps sharply → Blood diverted to skin for emergency cooling → Muscles & brain left short of O_2

Symptoms of dehydration can be diverse and encompass more than just thirst. The more prolonged or severe the dehydration, the more severe will be the symptoms. Ultimately, if dehydration remains untreated it can be fatal.

Dehydration Symptoms			
Early[25]	Prolonged[26]	Athletes[27]	Untreated[28]
Thirst	Very dark urine	Loss of performance	Delirium
Headache	Rapid breathing	Flushing	Extreme lethargy
General discomfort	Constipation	Low endurance	Seizures
Appetite loss	Hypotension	Rapid heart rate	Fainting
Dry skin	Dizziness	High body temp	Sunken eyes
Decreased urine	Fainting	Fatigue	Unconsciousness
Confusion	Listlessness		Swollen tongue
Tiredness	Insomnia		Death (extreme)
Irritability	Skin elasticity loss		

Blood Sugar Instability

Another common cause of fatigue is blood sugar instability. Maintenance of blood glucose levels under a variety of nutritional conditions and energetic demands lies at the heart of keeping energy levels stable and preventing fatigue. This is because it is the concentration of glucose in the blood that acts as the main control for the metabolic hormone *insulin*, which directs glucose to the cells to either be metabolised for energy or to be stored as fat. The ultimate consequence of failing to keep blood glucose in control is the development of *type 2 diabetes* (a form of diabetes mellitus).

Both increased blood glucose levels and diabetes are rising globally.[29] According to the World Health Authority (WHO), by 2030 approximately 366 million adults will have diabetes (with over 90% of these being type-2), which will result in diabetes being the seventh leading cause of death worldwide.[30] These are shocking statistics considering simple lifestyle measures have been shown to be effective in preventing or delaying the onset of type-2 diabetes.[31] It is perhaps no coincidence that this rise in blood sugar instability has also coincided with a rise in the numbers of people suffering fatigue.

Categories of Blood Sugar Instability

Blood sugar instability (without a diagnosis of diabetes) can be broadly classified into four different types:

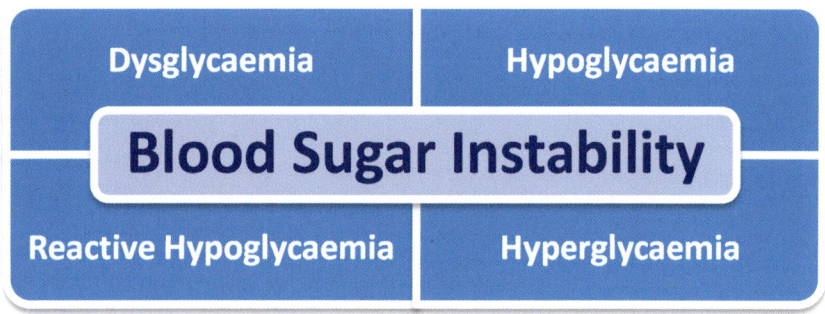

Dysglycaemia is often used to describe abnormal control of blood glucose levels when no firm diagnosis has been made. It refers to the fluctuation of blood sugar levels causing both **hypoglycaemia** and **hyperglycaemia.** It is heavily influenced by diet and the actions of the metabolic hormones *insulin* and *glucagon* and can have a direct effect on daily energy levels leading to feelings of fatigue. Medically, it is associated with diabetes but you can suffer from a 'sub-clinical' version, which often goes undetected by medical practitioners. In alternative medicine circles, this condition is often called **hypoglycaemia** or *"low blood sugar levels"*. It is commonly encountered through poor eating patterns and is often characterised by energy lows, shakiness, and altered mood and thinking, but without measured low glucose or risk of severe harm.

Dysglycaemia Symptoms[32]		
Fatigue	Poor stamina	Palpitations
Excessive sweating	Irritability	Anxiety/panic
Depression	Mood swings	Poor concentration
Headaches	Drowsiness	Clumsiness
Insomnia	Central fat deposition	Sweet cravings

Stimulant addictions	Alcoholism	Indigestion
PMS	Joint pain	Numbness
Hyperactivity	Nightmares	Breathlessness
Migraine	Vertigo	Muscular stiffness
Fainting	Stomach cramps	Cold extremities
Asthma	Allergies	Tinnitus

Hypoglycaemia literally means "low blood sugar". However, unlike dysglycaemia, this condition is a medical emergency that involves an abnormally diminished content of glucose in the blood.[33] It can produce a variety of symptoms and effects but the principal problems arise from an inadequate supply of glucose to the brain, resulting in impairment of function. Effects can range from feelings of discontentment, restlessness and malaise; to more serious issues such as seizures, unconsciousness, and (rarely) brain damage or death.

Hypoglycaemia Symptoms		
Shakiness	Anxiety	Nervousness
Palpitations	Tachycardia	Sweating
Coldness/clamminess	Dilated pupils	Hunger
Nausea/vomiting	Headache	Abdominal discomfort
Impaired judgment	Moodiness/Depression	Crying
Numbness/pins & needles	Irritability	Rage
Fatigue	Weakness	Lethargy
Sleepiness/insomnia	Confusion	Amnesia/memory loss
Dizziness	Blurred/double vision	Slurred speech
Ataxia/incoordination	Seizures	Coma

Not all of these symptoms occur in every case of hypoglycemia. There is no consistent order to their appearance, if symptoms even occur. Specific manifestations may also vary by age, severity of the hypoglycemia and the speed of the decline. The most common forms of hypoglycaemia occur as a complication of treatment of diabetes mellitus with insulin or oral medications. It is less common in non-diabetics but can occur at any age. In the non-diabetic individual, blood sugar disturbances are more likely to fall into the dysglycaemia category or the rarer reactive hypoglycaemia.

Reactive hypoglycaemia is a medical term describing recurrent episodes of symptomatic hypoglycaemia occurring within 4 hours[34] after a high carbohydrate meal in people who do not have diabetes. Hence, it is also called ***postprandial hypoglycaemia***. Medically, the prevalence of this condition is difficult to ascertain because the pattern of postprandial hypoglycaemia must meet the *Whipple triad criteria*[35] to be considered; whereby the hypoglycaemic symptoms correspond to measurably low blood glucose which is relieved by raising the glucose levels. Often, there is no official diagnosis. The symptoms, cause and treatment are usually similar to dysglycaemia.

Hyperglycaemia is commonly called "high blood sugar" and is a condition in which excessive amounts of glucose circulates in the blood. Temporary hyperglycemia, which often occurs in dysglycaemia, is often benign and asymptomatic. Blood glucose levels can rise well above normal for significant periods without producing any permanent effects or symptoms. However, chronic hyperglycemia - at levels more than slightly above normal - can produce a very wide variety of serious complications over a period of years, including damage to the kidneys, nerves, cardiovascular system, retina, feet and legs. Diabetes mellitus is by far the most common cause of chronic hyperglycemia, with treatment aimed at maintaining blood glucose at a level as close to normal as possible, in order to avoid these serious long-term complications.

Stress

Stress can have a major impact on energy levels. It comprises a complex series of physiologic and behavioural responses that aim to restore the challenged body to a state of equilibrium ***(homeostasis)***.[36] Factors that cause the body to diverge from homeostasis can range from physical events to psychological or anticipatory. The environment in which we live continually places demands upon us, both real and perceived, so the body needs to be able to adapt to these demands to function and survive. Hence, ***stress is the body's response to a challenge.***

The way in which it responds is to activate neuronal, hormonal and immune responses, which cause a number of physical changes that have both short and long-term effects. The actual process of trying to restore homeostasis consumes energy stores and nutrients, which can leave you energy and nutrient depleted.

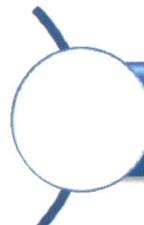

It is YOUR RESPONSE to stress rather than the size of the actual stress that is IMPORTANT.

The intensity and duration of the stress can also change depending upon your circumstances and your emotional condition.[37] **Acute stress** tends to have short-term effects; whereas **chronic stress** can have long-term effects that can impair your ability to adapt, which in turn will affect your mental and physical wellbeing. There are a whole range of stress factors, many of which are not commonly associated with stress by the average person. Those factors can be environmental or emotional, and can involve external and internal stimuli.

Stress Factors			
Internal Stimuli	**External Stimuli**	**Social**	**Life Experiences**
Fatigue	Temperature	Relationship conflict	Poverty
Hunger	Seasonal changes	Break-ups	Unemployment
Thirst	Sight/light	Birth	Depression
Pain	Smell	Death	Obsessive disorder
Thoughts/images	Hearing/noise	Marriage	Heavy drinking
Perceived stress	Touch	Divorce	Work pressure
Sleep disturbances	Taste	Deception	Exams
Fear/worry	Air/water quality	Housing	Immobility/injury

Stress symptoms can also be multiple and vague and can often overlap with symptoms of blood sugar instability. Symptoms may be cognitive, emotional, physical, behavioural or a combination of disturbances on multiple levels.

Stress Symptoms			
Cognitive	**Emotional**	**Physical**	**Behavioural**
Forgetfulness	Moodiness	Aches and pains	Eating more/less
Poor concentration	Irritability	Diarrhoea/constipation	Sleep disturbances
Poor judgment	Agitation	Urination frequency	Social withdrawal
Pessimistic	Inability to relax	Indigestion	Procrastination
Anxiety	Overwhelmed	Nausea/dizziness	Neglect
Worry	Loneliness/isolation	Sugar cravings	Stimulant use
Negative	Depression	Rapid heartbeat	Nervous habits
Critical	Unhappiness	Frequent colds	Short temper
Judgmental	Anger/rage	Loss of sex drive	Personality change
Racing thoughts	Tearfulness	Irregular periods	Alcohol/smoking

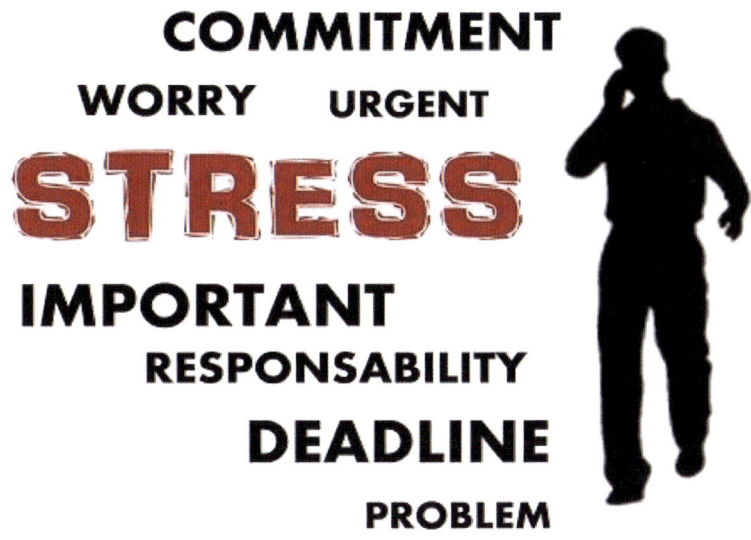

Source: www.pixabay.com

General Adaptation Syndrome

The physiology of stress is characterised by the **General Adaptation Syndrome (GAS)** - as conceptualised by the pioneering endocrinologist *Hans Selye*.[38] This characterises a universal non-specific stress response consisting of three specific physiological stages.

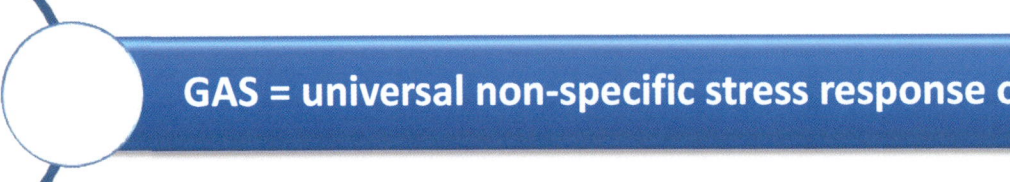
GAS = universal non-specific stress response of 3 stages

The first stage is the *alarm stage,* which is the shock phase and promotes nervous system activity to mobilise resources. Here, resistance to stress drops below normal and the body's 'fight or flight' hormones (*adrenaline and nor-adrenaline*) respond to stress. The second stage is the *resistance stage*, where the body mounts a systemic response via the hormone *cortisol* to increase energy levels to try and adapt to the stress. The third and final stage is *recovery OR exhaustion.* In the *recovery stage*, the hormonal compensatory mechanisms have overcome the stress. However, if the stress is not overcome, the *exhaustion stage* will prevail. This is where resources are so depleted that abnormal function occurs and stress symptoms re-appear. Illness may result.

Alarm
- **Shock** – resistance to stress drops below normal.
- **Fight-or-flight** – *neuro-hormones* respond to stress.

Resistance
- **Systemic response** – *cortisol* increases energy levels.
- **Adaptation** – body adapts but resources depleted.

Recovery
- **Compensation mechanisms** – overcome stressor.
- **High blood glucose levels** – used for regeneration

OR

Exhaustion
- **Resources depleted** – abnormal function.
- **Stress symptoms** – reappear. Illness may result.

In the shock phase of the response, stress symptoms will become apparent. During the resistance or adaptation stage, symptoms can often disappear as the body mobilises resources to adapt to the stressor. This stage can last for a long-time depending upon the individual and the situation. Ultimately, if the stressor continues for a long period, as with chronic stress, or multiple stressors overwhelm the body's resources, then the exhaustion stage will ensue. This uniform pattern of resistance to stress can be illustrated by the *general adaptation curve:*

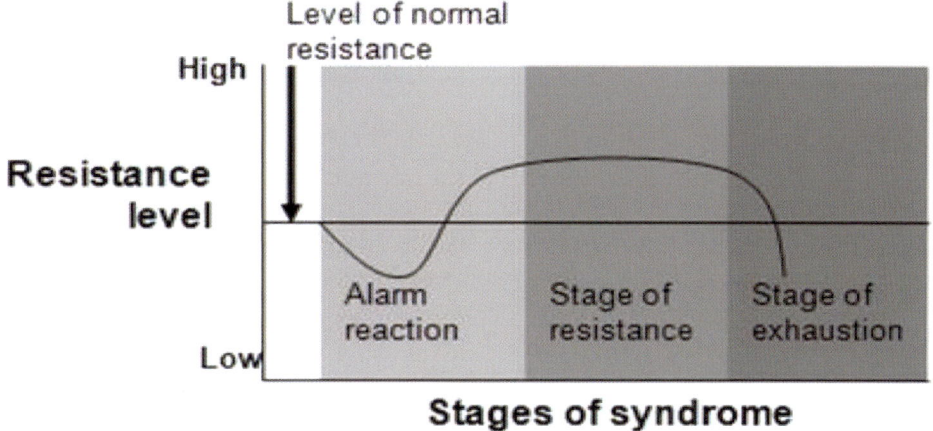

Source: www.ukessays.com

It is the exhaustion stage that is also called **adrenal fatigue** by alternative medicine practitioners. This is because the hormones involved in the stress response (**adrenaline, nor-adrenaline** and **cortisol**) are produced by the adrenal glands and these become disturbed through over-stimulation. Despite *Hans Selye* profoundly influencing the scientific study of stress through his well-publicised research in the early twentieth century,[39] general medicine is still very slow (if at all) to acknowledge that the non-specific symptoms or illnesses that occur as a result of stress are indeed stress related. Furthermore, many medical practitioners do not take seriously any suggestion of "adrenal exhaustion", even though the WHO formally recognised this condition in 2010.[40] Yet it is very real condition that appears more and more frequently and can significantly impair the lifestyle of those affected.

Chronic Fatigue Syndrome (CFS)

CFS is the common name[41] for a group of significantly debilitating medical conditions characterised by persistent fatigue and other specific symptoms that lasts for a minimum of six months in adults (and 3 months in children or adolescents).[42] It may also be referred to as *myalgic encephalomyelitis (ME)* or *post-viral fatigue syndrome (PVFS)* as it is often triggered by viral infection. ***The fatigue is not due to exertion, not significantly relieved by rest, and is not caused by other medical conditions.***[43]

Although the aetiology of CFS is not fully understood it is believed to have multiple causes.[44] Dr. Sarah Myhill[45] - a leading UK authority on CFS - believes that the syndrome is a stress-induced disorder leading to poor energy delivery at the cellular level. She defines stress as including infectious, physical, mental and emotional stress. As part of the general response to stress, Dr. Myhill regards the **adrenal glands** as being centrally important and cites the well-illustrated work of *Hans Selye*. The key dysfunction appears to be that the body is required to generate energy faster than it can supply it, hence fatigue being the main symptom of the condition.

CFS Symptoms[46]		
Severe fatigue	Malaise after exertion	Mental/physical exhaustion
Sleep disturbances	Insomnia	Unrefreshing sleep
Severe headaches	Cognitive difficulties	Depression
Muscular/joint pain	Muscle weakness	Poor stamina
Light/noise/smell sensitivity	Alcohol/food sensitivity	Digestive disturbances
Sore throat	Swollen lymph nodes	Respiratory problems

CFS recognition has come a long way since the 1980s when it was termed *"Yuppie flu"* and ascribed to a psychological problem rather than a physical one. However, there are some doctors in the medical community who still do not recognise it as a real condition, nor is their agreement on its prevalence; though it is generally agreed that it affects more women than men.[47] As a consequence, many people can suffer from a life-debilitating condition for many years without getting the help they need. However, a ray of hope for such sufferers can now be found in the recent recognition that too much emphasis has previously been placed on psychological research and insufficient attention to biomedical research; and that it is further biomedical research that is now required to help discover a cause and more effective management for the condition.[48]

Chapter 4: Medical Management

Fatigue

Fatigue is reported as the main presenting symptom in up to 10% of all patients who see a doctor.[49] Both its non-specific nature and its high prevalence make it a challenging problem for GPs to manage. The symptom may indicate a wide range of conditions, including respiratory, cardiovascular, endocrine, gastrointestinal, haematological, infectious, neurological and musculoskeletal, mood disorders, sleep disorders and cancer.[50] Also, its prevalence is highest in those with chronic disease.[51] Regardless of the underlying pathology, fatigue has social, physiological and psychological dimensions.[52]

The goal of the doctor is to identify and rule out any treatable conditions. This is generally done by considering your medical history, any other symptoms that are present and evaluating the qualities of fatigue itself. Sleep patterns, stress, depression and psychological conditions, drug abuse, poor diet and lack of physical exercise (which paradoxically can increase fatigue) will all be routinely screened. Basic medical tests may also be performed to rule out other common causes of fatigue. These include blood tests to check for infection or anaemia; a urinalysis to look for signs of liver disease or diabetes mellitus; and other tests to check for kidney and liver function, such as a comprehensive metabolic panel.[53] More specific tests may include an HIV test or pregnancy test.

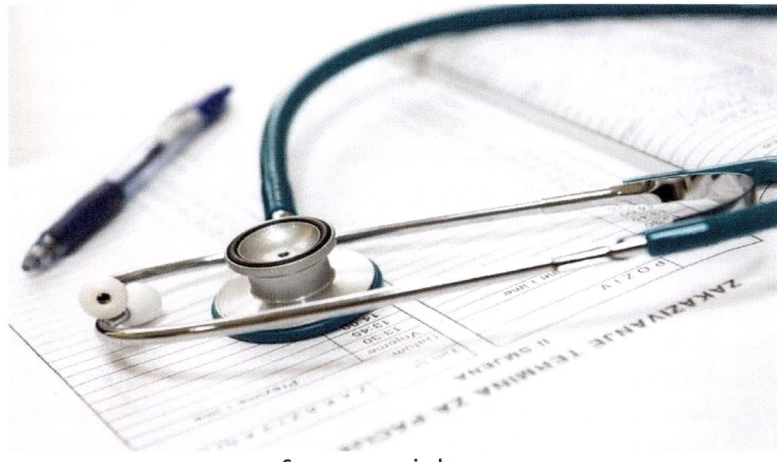

Source: www.pixabay.com

Despite all of these tests, a recent study concluded that only about 50% of people who have fatigue receive a diagnosis that could explain the fatigue after a year with the condition.[54] In those people who have a possible diagnosis, musculoskeletal (19.4%) and psychological problems (16.5%) are the most common. Definitive physical conditions were only found in 8.2% of cases.[55] This leaves a staggering 50% of fatigue sufferers with no explanation as to the reason for their condition and without a treatment plan to help them overcome the problem. No wonder more and more people are turning to alternative health in an attempt to relieve their fatigue symptoms.

Dehydration

The treatment for minor dehydration is drinking water and stopping fluid loss. Plain water restores only the blood volume, which inhibits the thirst mechanism before solute levels can be replenished.[56] In more severe cases, correction of a dehydrated state is accomplished by the replenishment of necessary water and electrolytes (minerals that help to regulate water balance and cell function), either orally or intravenously. As oral rehydration is less painful, invasive, and expensive; and easier to provide; it is the treatment of choice for mild dehydration. Intravenous rehydration, however, may be necessary in severe cases where fainting, unconsciousness or other severely inhibiting symptom is present. Complete resolution is normal in all but the most extreme cases.

Blood Sugar Instability

Reactive hypoglycaemia - The U.S. National Institute of Health (NIH) recommends dietary intervention in the first instance and advocates the following:[57]

1.	Eat small meals and snacks about every 3 hours.
2.	Avoid or limit sugar intake, including high sugar drinks and alcohol.
3.	Exercise regularly.
4.	Eat a variety of foods, including protein, whole-grains, fruits and vegetables.
5.	Choose high-fibre foods.
6.	Follow a low-carbohydrate diet.

To confirm a diagnosis, a doctor can administer an **HbA1c** (glycated haemoglobin) test to measure the blood sugar average over the past 2–3 months. Additionally, a 6-hour glucose tolerance test will chart blood sugar during the past six hours. A blood glucose level below 70 mg/dL (3.9 mmol/L) at the time of symptoms, followed by relief after eating confirms a diagnosis for reactive hypoglycemia.[58]

Hypoglycaemia - is treated by restoring the blood glucose level to normal by the ingestion or administration of dextrose or carbohydrate foods. Blood glucose can be raised to normal within minutes by taking (or receiving) 10-20 g of carbohydrate,[59] either via food or drink. This equates to approximately either 100–120 ml of orange, apple, or grape juice; 120-150 ml of regular (non-diet) soda; or 1 slice of bread, or 4 crackers, or about 1 serving of most starchy foods. Symptoms should begin to improve within 5 minutes, though full recovery may take 10–20 minutes. In more severe circumstances, it is treated by injection or infusion of *glucagon* (a metabolic hormone). Recurrent hypoglycemia may be prevented by reversing or removing the underlying cause; by increasing the frequency of meals; with medications like diazoxide, octreotide, or glucocorticoids (adrenal hormones); or by surgical removal of much of the pancreas.

Stress

Primary care settings will generally recommend stress reduction techniques to help you cope and manage your stress. These can include exercise; nutrition; techniques on relaxation, time-management and mindfulness; social support and cognitive-behaviour therapy (CBT).[60] GPs can recommend stress management groups or classes, some of which are run in doctor's surgeries or community centres. If these stress management techniques do not work, referral can be made to professionals, such as social workers, psychologists, and psychiatrists. Where stress is causing serious health problems, such as high blood pressure, you may be recommended medication or further tests.

Chronic Fatigue Syndrome

The therapeutic approach to CFS is complex and requires a combination of different therapeutic treatments. Although many therapies for CFS have been examined, cognitive-behaviour therapy (CBT), together with gradual physical exercise, has proven to be the most effective.[61] CBT is a type of therapy that aims to change the way you think, feel and behave. A 2008 review found that 40% of patients reported fatigue improvements after CBT.[62] Many drug therapies have also been used for treatment, although the quality of the available evidence is poor,[63] so medication plays a minor role in CFS management.[64] For those people in pain or having trouble sleeping, the anti-depressant drug *amitriptyline* is sometimes used. Many people do not fully recover from CFS even with treatment.[65] Hence, there is a clear need for finding a better therapeutic approach for CFS sufferers.

Chapter 5: Pathophysiology

Energy Demand

You have a constant need for energy to fuel your bodily functions and sustain your survival. The energy that you require can be divided into two parts:

Energy Requirements
1. Basal *(lowest possible level)* metabolic requirements.
2. Energy required for activity, including brain (20%) activity.

The **basal metabolic rate (BMR)** is defined as the rate that heat is eliminated from the body at rest when the temperature is normal. Essentially, **this refers to the rate at which you burn your fuel**. An average person requires approximately 2,000-2,400 calories per day, although a large man doing heavy physical work may require up to 6,000 calories per day.[66] However, these requirements can vary from individual to individual and do not take into account *environmental factors* that can significantly impact on energy requirements. Environmental factors can include all the stress factors previously identified; as well as a cold/hot environment (which can increase the BMR rate by 5-20% to correct body temperature) and physical activity or the lack of it, which can increase or decrease energy requirements.

Cellular Energy Production

Biological energy production (AKA *metabolism*) occurs at the cellular level via a process called *cellular respiration*. This encompasses two sets of metabolic reactions and processes that allow for energy production with or without the presence of oxygen. The main process is *aerobic respiration,* which requires oxygen to function. However, in the absence of insufficient oxygen (such as with intense exercise) it is very important that the body is still able to generate energy, and so it switches to *anaerobic respiration*, which does not require oxygen.

Aerobic Respiration	• Requires oxygen
Anaerobic Respiration	• Does not require oxygen

Through these processes, enzymes catalyse the transformation of energy from food into biological energy - *adenosine triphosphate (ATP)* - via the coupling and uncoupling of one of the phosphate molecules of the ATP molecule. The rate at which this transformation takes place is called the *metabolic rate* or the speed of metabolism.

Cellular Respiration

Aerobic respiration takes place in three stages:

	Aerobic Respiration	
1.	**Glycolysis**	Glucose is partially broken down into **pyruvate** inside the cell cytosol to produce **2 ATP molecules**.
2	**Krebs Cycle** (AKA Citric Acid Cycle)	The 2 ATP molecules from glycolysis feed into a complicated set of reactions inside the **mitochondria** (*organelles inside of the cell*) to produce **2 ATP molecules**.
3	**Electron Transport Chain**	By-products of the Krebs cycle then feed into another series of reactions inside of the mitochondria to produce **32 - 38 ATP molecules**.

Oxygen is necessary in both the Krebs Cycle and the Electron Transport Chain as it combines with hydrogen to form water, which prevents the build-up of electrons (the electrons being the energy transfer carriers).

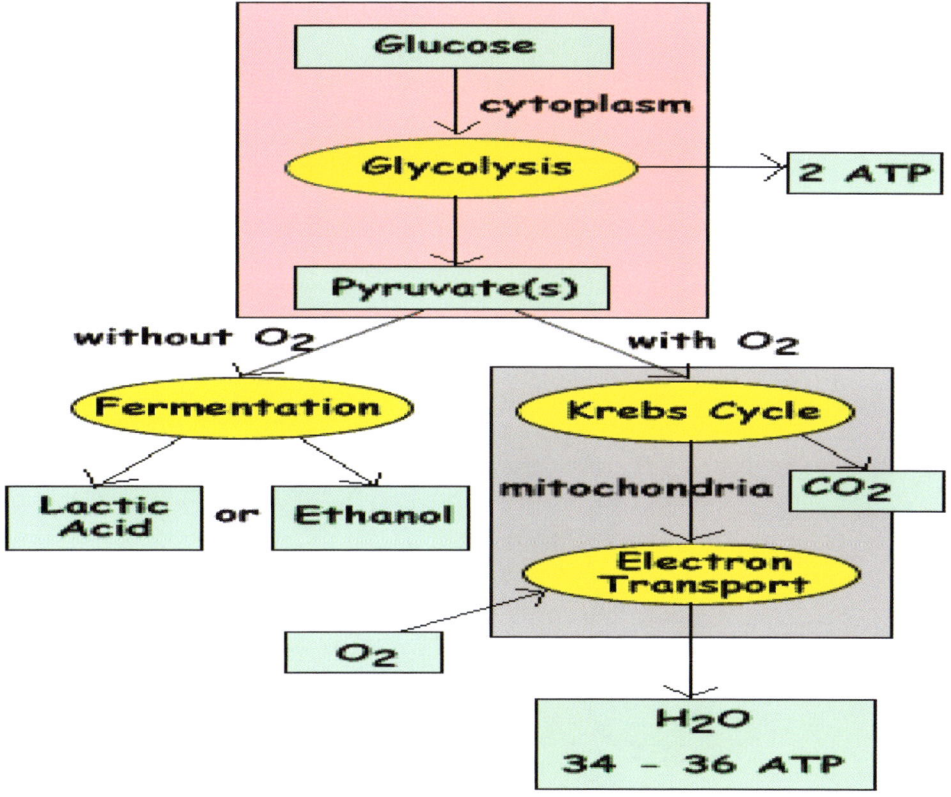

Source: www.room114wikispaces.com

Anaerobic respiration generates ATP energy without oxygen. Here, pyruvate is not transported into the mitochondria but undergoes fermentation in the cytosol (cell fluid) to lactic acid and alcohol. When oxygen becomes available, the lactic acid molecule can be re-converted to ATP, which is then re-directed back through to the Krebs Cycle and Electron Transport Chain pathway. Anaerobic respiration is less efficient at using energy than aerobic respiration because the waste products of lactic acid and alcohol contain potential energy that is released when oxygen becomes available. However, it is a very important process that enables energy to be produced when there is insufficient oxygen, such as with intense exercise or at high altitudes.

Circadian Regulation

The actual process of energy production is governed by a regular **circadian cycle**[67] - a biological process that repeats over a 24-hour period (similar to a sleep/wake cycle). The rhythm of this circadian cycle is driven by a group of genes called ***clock genes***. There are multiple clock genes found throughout the body, especially in peripheral tissues such as the liver, fat, muscle, heart and blood vessels.[68] However, they are all regulated by the *master clock,* which is called the "**pacemaker**" and resides in the **suprachiasmatic nucleus (SCN)** of the **hypothalamus** (the area in the brain that links the nervous system to the endocrine system). The SCN synchronises internal biological processes to external time cues by activating the hypothalamus,[69] which disseminates the signal to other parts of the body through hormones such as cortisol (stress hormone) and melatonin (sleep promoter).[70]

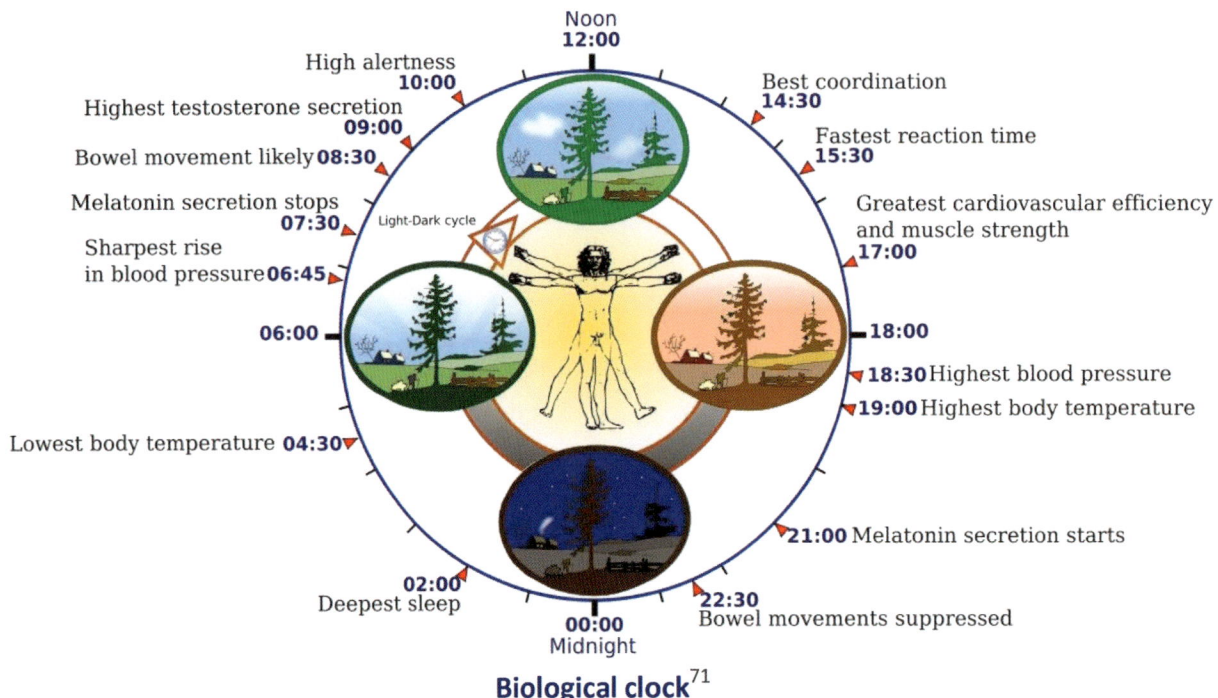

Biological clock[71]

External factors that affect hormone production can compromise the clock function, such as a high-fat diet, obesity, jetlag, shift-work and sleep disruption.[72] These factors could explain why the effects of our modern 24/7 lifestyles can disrupt our natural rhythms, which in turn can significantly affect health and disease.[73] Disrupted circadian rhythms has now been found to be an exacerbating factor in ***metabolic syndrome***[74] – a disorder of energy utilisation and storage that encompasses abdominal obesity and elevated blood pressure, blood sugar and cholesterol. These are all conditions that are approaching epidemic levels in modern society.

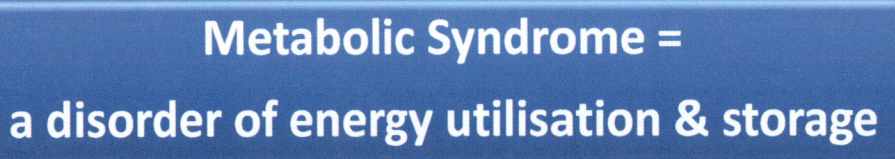

Metabolic Syndrome = a disorder of energy utilisation & storage

Nervous System Regulation

A central neural circuitry is also involved in the homeostatic regulation of nutrient and energy intake,[75] and is influenced by environmental cues[76] such as hedonism, reward and memory representations of food experiences.[77] This neural processing occurs in the brain via a two–step process that involves integration of sensory information from the *hypothalamus* and input from the motivational system in the *cortico-limbic system*.

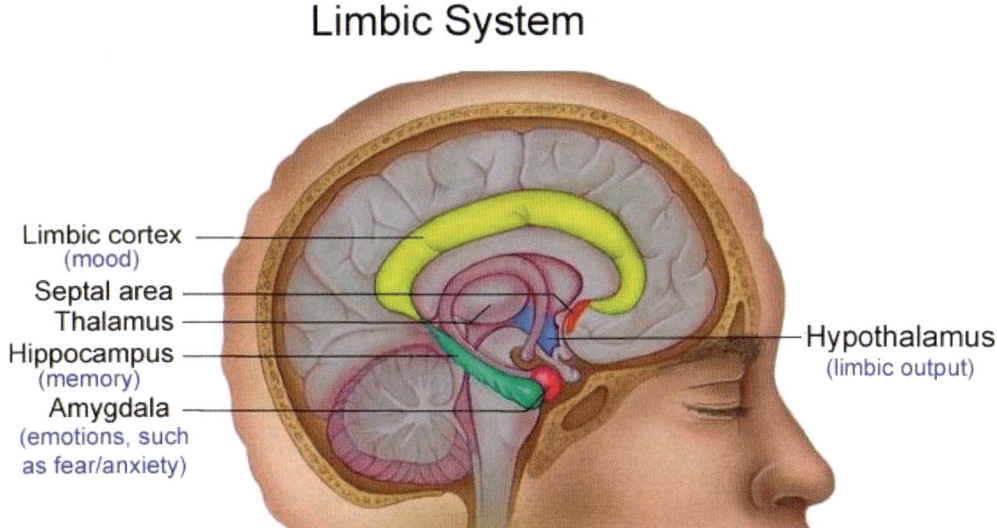

Source: www.conwaypsychology.webs.com

Brain Neural Processing	
1. **Sensory Information**	Satiety or hunger signals are sent to the *hypothalamus* via sensory neurons, which determines the hunger drive.[78]
2 **The Motivational System**	The *cortico-limbic system* is engaged to find and eat food that generates a reward and gratification feeling.[79] This reward system takes into account the sight, smell and taste of food (as well as metabolites and hormones) to rely on earlier food experiences that are stored as 'food memories'.[80]

This same basic two-step neural processing may also be responsible for the homeostatic-like regulation of individual nutrients.[81] The difference being that instead of trying to satisfy a general energy deficit, the system satisfies nutrient-specific appetites. Hence, this pathway could account for the expression of the *'wisdom of the body'*, whereby you crave a particular food that contains a nutrient that your body is lacking.

Hormone Regulation

The endocrine system is intricately involved in energy homeostasis through its regulation of fuel delivery and the rate of energy production.

Key Hormonal Regulators		
Hormone	Origin	Function
1. Insulin & Glucagon	Pancreas	Fuel delivery to cells for energy or storage.
2. Cortisol	Adrenal Glands	Increase fuel supply.
3. Thyroxine	Thyroid Gland	Increase rate of fuel burning.

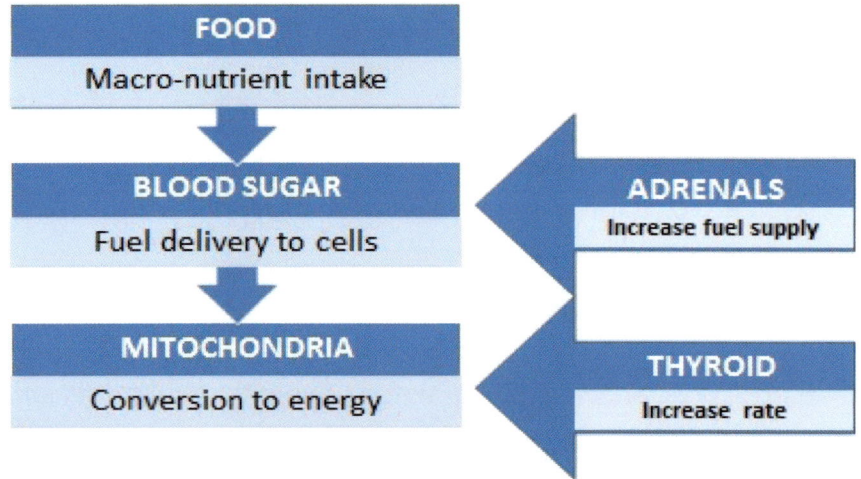

Pancreatic Hormones

Insulin and **glucagon** play central and opposing roles in maintaining blood sugar levels and fuel delivery through regulation of nutrient storage and availability – insulin lowers blood glucose levels, whilst glucagon raises them. In the *fed state*, insulin stimulates the transport of glucose into cells to either be consumed as fuel for energy or to be stored short-term as glycogen (in the liver and muscles) or long-term as fat (in the fat cells). In the *fasting state*, insulin secretion decreases and glucagon secretion increases. Glucagon breaks down stored energy supplies – first glycogen, then protein and fat – to release glucose into the blood to be used as fuel for energy. This glucose transport system becomes impaired when there is insulin deficiency or when the cells become non-responsive to insulin (*insulin resistance*) and can lead to *diabetes mellitus* (high blood sugar levels).

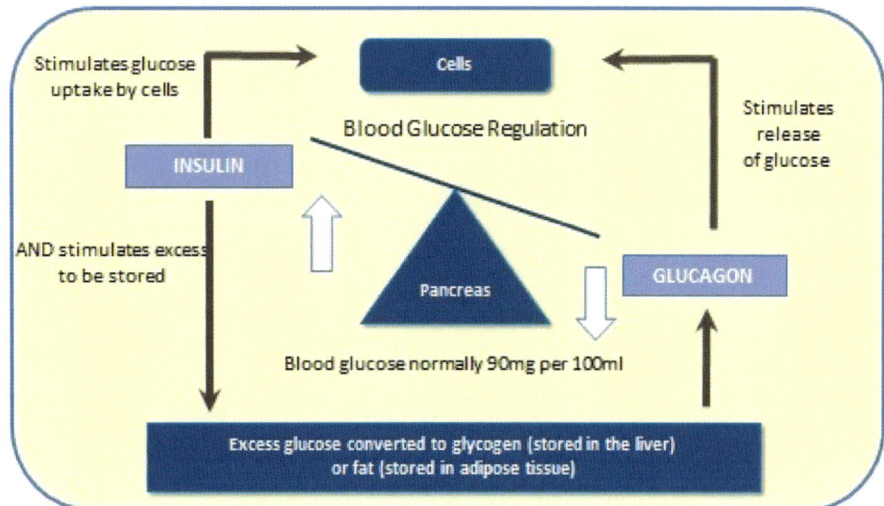

BioCare (2014) Energy in Practice

Adrenal Hormones

The adrenal glands (which sit at the top of the kidneys) act as a **critical energy back-up system** and are integrally involved in energy production through the management of the stress response. During times of stress or when blood sugar levels drop too low (which in itself is a stressor), the adrenal hormones **adrenaline** (AKA epinephrine) and **nor-adrenaline** (AKA nor-epinephrine) are largely responsible for the immediate reactions through nervous system activation, which trigger a burst of energy for a 'fight or flight' situation. **Cortisol** then mobilises nutrient stores by increasing *gluconeogenesis* (glucose generation from non-carbohydrate substances) and triggering *glucagon* secretion to break down glycogen and fat stores. This increases the blood levels of glucose and fatty acids, which are then used as fuel for energy production.

Adrenal disruption occurs when the adrenal response to stressors is compromised, resulting in an abnormal balance of cortisol. As a generalisation, adrenal stress can begin with excess cortisol secretion; progress to a pattern of 'inverted' secretion (whereby cortisol is low in the morning and then increases during the day through use of stimulants); and eventually lead to complete adrenal exhaustion. Intermittent fatigue and irritability are symptoms of excess cortisol, whereas fatigue that increases through the day is a symptom of low cortisol and fatigue unrelieved by rest is symptomatic of adrenal exhaustion.

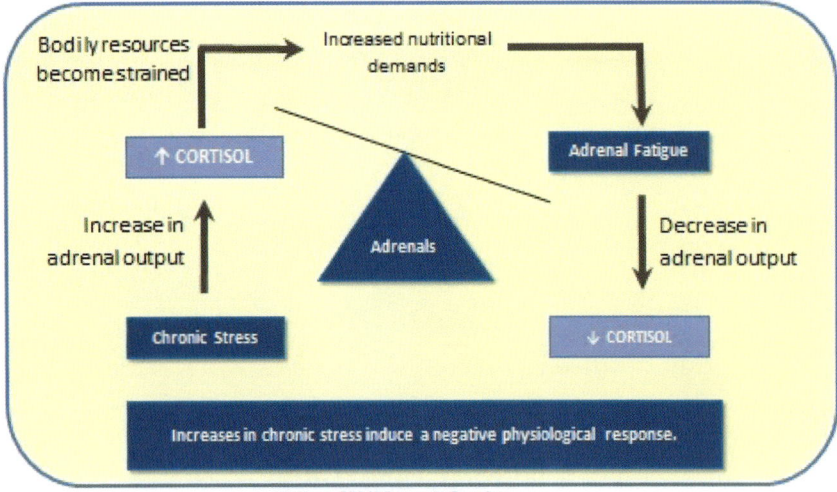

BioCare (2014) Energy in Practice

Thyroid Hormones

The thyroid gland (found in the neck) is one of the largest endocrine glands in the body. It produces two principal hormones: **triiodothyronine (T_3)** and **thryoxine (T_4)**, which control how quickly energy is used. These hormones regulate metabolism by altering mitochondrial ATP production through influencing oxygen consumption and nutrient utilisation.[82] They can alter the BMR by as much as 50% in either direction.

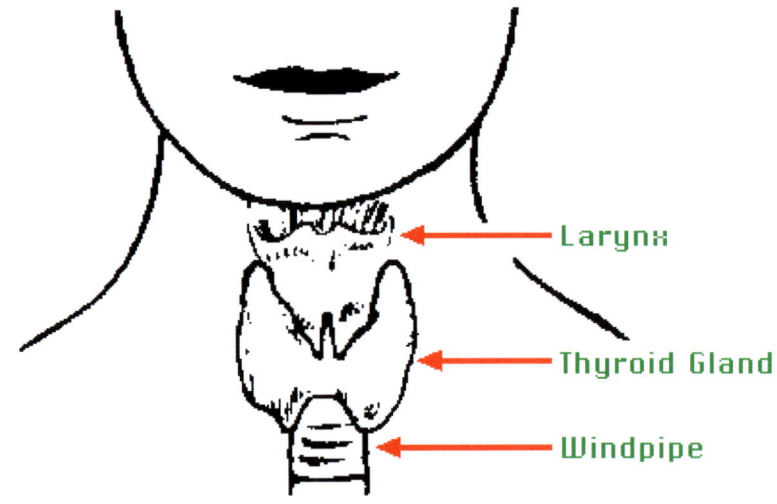

Source: www.macaperu.com

Dysfunctional thyroid production has profound alterations on energy homeostasis at many levels, including glucose uptake and production, as well as fat breakdown.[83] It can also lead to the clinically recognised conditions **hypothyroidism** (low hormone output) and **hyperthyroidism** (excessive hormone output). Hypothyroidism is the most common and can produce a range of symptoms, whilst hyperthyroidism is much less common and is mainly associated with the autoimmune condition Grave's disease.[84]

Hypothyroidism Symptoms		
Low energy	Mental fatigue	Stubborn weight gain
Low body temperature	Dry and scaly skin	Thinning hair & eyebrows
Brittle nails	Vocal hoarseness	

Around 4.6% of the US population has hypothyroidism.[85] However, it is projected that 12% of the population will go on to develop a thyroid condition during their lifetime, although 60% of those will be unaware of their condition.[86] A similar picture has emerged in the UK.[87] What is becoming clear is that dysfunctional thyroid hormone production is linked to the **metabolic syndrome.** Shocking statistics indicate that a quarter of the world's adults have metabolic syndrome.[88]

Brain Regulatory Control

The brain has now emerged as the crucial regulator of whole-body energy homeostasis via a complex neuroendocrine system,[89][90] which receives and integrates a variety of signals regarding energy status that promotes or limits food intake.[91] Central to this regulation is the **arcuate nucleus (ARC)** of the hypothalamus, which senses and integrates hormonal, neural and energy substrate signals.[92] These include appetite regulating hormones – ghrelin (the 'hunger' hormone) and leptin (the 'satiety' hormone) – as well as insulin, thyroid hormones,[93] and glucose-sensing neurons.[94] Together, these signals provide information about energy status[95] that allows the brain to promote or limit food intake to regulate energy balance.

Energy balance is highly regulated

Chapter 6: Clinical Considerations

Where to Start?

Knowing where to start can be challenging, if not overwhelming. Regulatory control is complex, whilst there is great potential for disruption from an array of factors. However, there are a number of common features that can be taken into consideration when addressing energy levels.

Energy Disturbances – Clinical Considerations	
Stress	Inflammation
Blood Sugar Control	Thyroid Imbalance
Gastrointestinal Tract Imbalance	Mitochondrial Dysfunction
Adrenal Overstimulation	Environmental Toxic Exposure

Stress

Stress is so pervasive in today's society and is so integral to energy demand and supply that it often lays at the heart of the matter. It plays a part in regulating appetite and storing fat through neuronal stimulation of the appetite-satiety centres in the hypothalamus.[96] During *acute stress*, the nerve messenger **neuropeptide Y (NPY)** is inhibited leading to reduced food intake and fat storage; whereas during *chronic/repeated stress*, NPY release is increased leading to greater food ingestion and fat storage,[97] especially as abdominal fat.[98] This increased food intake diminishes the stress response,[99] which is why you often feel better after eating.

Acute Stress	• Reduced food intake and fat storage
Chronic Stress	• Increased food intake and fat storage

Chronic stress also promotes unhealthy behaviours such as a sedentary lifestyle, alcohol consumption and smoking;[100] whilst food ingestion to relieve anxiety is a harmful coping strategy and can lead to undesirable weight gain and obesity.[101] It is always necessary to consider your stress levels and determine where your stress is actually coming from. Many people simply don't realise that they are under stressful conditions. Undertaking a comprehensive audit of your lifestyle will highlight situations that are leading to an energy drain.

Blood Sugar Control

As the fuel delivery system of the body, blood glucose regulation is central to energy balance. However, today's diet is far removed from that of our ancestors and this has had a profound effect on blood sugar control. In the last 100 years, rapid changes in the Western diet through the advent of modern farming and food processing have changed what we eat, when we eat and how we eat. *"Fast food"* - which packs palatable food into convenient servings that can be prepared and eaten quickly - is popular across Europe and North America. Such foods are high in energy and fat but low in fibre and nutrients;[102] which is markedly different from the historical low-energy-density diet that the human gut was adapted to over several millennia.[103] This fast food type diet produces lower satiety signals,[104] and leads to over-eating, fast-absorption of glucose into the blood and erratic blood sugar levels. Going back to basics with your diet is absolutely essential to rebalance your energy levels.

The Gastrointestinal (GI) Tract

The GI tract is the main organ responsible for the intake and absorption of food. Hence, it is not surprising that it plays a role in appetite regulation.[105] Such appetite control regulates the delivery of nutrients to the blood and occurs via nutrient and neural stimulation, as well as gut hormone production. The major gut hormones are **ghrelin** (*the hunger hormone*) which is produced in the stomach[106] when the stomach is empty to initiate meal intake;[107] and **peptide YY (PYY)** and **glucagon-like peptide-1 (GLP-1),** which affect gastric motility.[108] Production of these hormones cause a decrease in gastric emptying, which reduces food intake, slows small-intestinal transit time,[109] and increases absorption.[110] This appetite-suppressing gut hormone signalling is heavily influenced via the effects of diet on the gut micro-flora.[111]

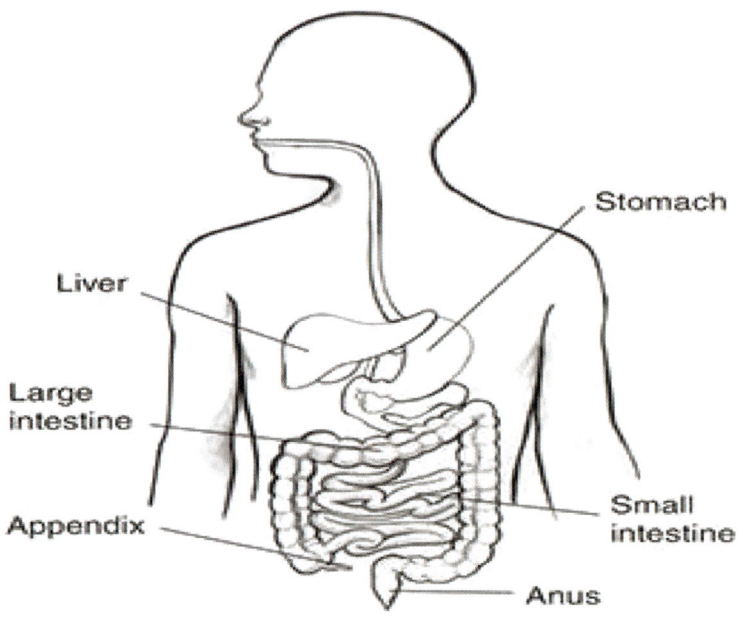
Source: www.exeterhospital.com

It is now recognised that there is a connection between gut flora, energy production and metabolic-related disorders.[112] Changes in the gut microbiota are correlated with the development of obesity, insulin resistance and diabetes.[113] The microflora have been found to play an important role in weight regulation through their involvement with appetite control[114] Modulation of their composition with **probiotics** (live bacteria) stimulates the production of the gut hormone **GLP-1**,[115] resulting in reduced food intake and improved glucose tolerance.[116]

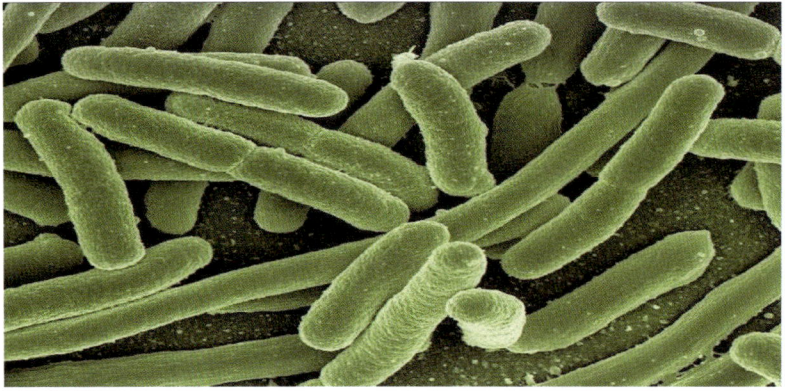
Source: www.pixabay.com

Diet is one of the most pivotal factors in the development of gut flora from infancy to old age.[117] A high consumption of fat and a low intake of fibre, fruits, vegetables and meat are associated with decreased microbial diversity.[118] As we age, life changes can also impact on the gut microbial population. These include physiological changes, dietary choices, use of antibiotics and prescription drugs, and living situation (community-dwelling, hospitalisation, long-term care).[119] Stress also significantly impacts the gut by altering *gut-brain interactions* that lead to alterations in gut microflora, inflammation and stress-associated gastrointestinal disorders.[120]

The gut is your body's interface with contents from the external environment. As such, a **gut-brain axis** exists whereby the peripheral and central systems link and feedback to each other continuously to control energy homeostasis.[121] This crosstalk allows you to adapt to changes in the environment and to ensure that energy is constantly available for your needs. Your perception of hunger and satiety is modulated through this network depending upon energy status, environmental stimuli, as well as other needs and behaviours.[122] Ongoing active research into the gut-brain axis[123] in the development of therapies against metabolic disorders[124] is highlighting the importance of the gut in relation to energy metabolism. Consequently, strategies to improve gut health should always be considered.

Adrenal Over-Stimulation

Any type of stress will involve stimulation of the adrenal glands as they are integral to the *stress-response mechanism* (termed the **hypothalamic-pituitary-adrenal (HPA) axis)**.[125] Stress in itself is advantageous to our survival because it leads to a specific cluster of time-limited, behavioural and physical changes that allow us to deal with emergency situations[126] and a constantly changing environment.[127] However, when stress becomes prolonged without resolution through repeated stressors, this can disrupt the pathways involved in metabolism, growth, reproduction, immunity, personality and behaviour.[128] This, in turn, can then lead to a wide range of health conditions, including severe fatigue.[129]

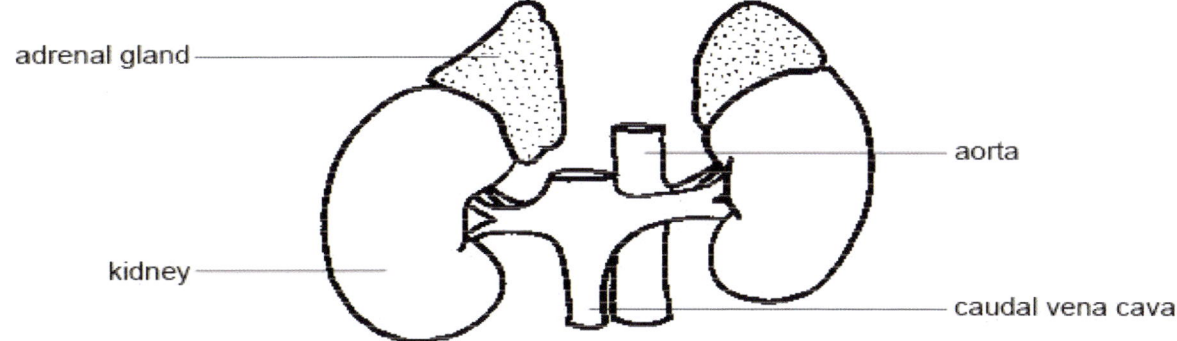

Source: www.en.wikibooks.org

HPA axis activation promotes a redirection of energy, in order to deliver oxygen and nutrients to organs and tissues involved in the stress response.[130] It also temporarily suppresses other non-emergency functions, such as digestion, reproduction, growth, and overall immunity.[131] All of these acute effects increase the capacity for energy generation over a limited period of time to improve your 'fight or flight ability'.[132] Cortisol is the final mediator of HPA axis activation and is the main adrenal hormone, playing a key role in modulating the stress response.[133] However, with over-stimulation through chronic stress,[134] it can be potentially damaging.

Chronic cortisol exposure can dysregulate multiple metabolic pathways[135] and shift metabolism from an *anabolic* (growth) to a *catabolic* (breaking-down) state.[136] This redistributes fat from peripheral tissues to central deposition and increases the size and number of fat cells.[137] It also enhances consumption of high fat and highly palatable foods,[138] decreases energy expenditure[139] and diminishes satiety signals.[140] These changes lead to a progressive increase in central fat, hyperglycemia, dyslipidemia, hypertension, insulin resistance[141] and metabolic disorders.[142][143] Hence, where stress is an issue, there is a need to remove the stressor(s), as well as provide additional specific nutrients to support the requirements for increased energy generation.

Inflammation

Stress also leads to the secretion of **inflammatory mediators** - molecules released by immune cells during times of possible harm - which can activate the HPA axis.[144] Although inflammation is part of the normal immune response – it induces pain, swelling, redness and warmth to promote healing after injury – it needs to be switched off after healing has occurred to prevent damage[145] **Cortisol is the main anti-inflammatory of the body that switches off the inflammation**[146] and regulates up to 2,000 genes involved in the immune system.[147] However, chronic stress blunts the effect of cortisol leading to increased inflammation.[148] Inflammation has been shown to be involved in the development of metabolic disturbances,[149] whilst uncontrolled inflammation is a key pathogenic mechanism in many diseases.[150]

The effects of stress on the inflammatory response occur in three stages,[151] with the second and third stage responses being equated to "systemic low grade inflammation":[152]

Stress and the Inflammatory Response[153]	
1. Early Stage	Down-regulation of pro-inflammatory mediators and up-regulation of anti-inflammatory mediators.
2. Sustained Stress	Blunted stress response, reduced immune sensitivity to cortisol and up-regulation of pro-inflammatory mediators.
3. HPA Axis Fatigue	Increased pro-inflammatory mediators, inflammation, and possible disease.

This increased inflammation can induce a re-allocation of energy directed towards the activated immune system – and requiring a similar amount of energy as that of the brain and muscles.[154] There is also a rapid increase in thyroid hormone production (to increase the rate of energy production), followed by a rapid down-regulation of thyroid hormone production;[155] leading to altered thyroid hormone production and metabolic disturbance. This association between low-grade inflammation and disturbed metabolism is also linked to obesity (which is now considered a state of chronic low-grade inflammation)[156] and shows how important it is to address inflammation as standard practice in improving metabolic balance.

Thyroid Imbalance

In virtually any type of situation characterized by an increased secretion of cortisol, altered thyroid hormone production and metabolism occurs, even when changes in the cortisol levels are within the normal range.[157] Significantly, the metabolism of those hormones - which is critical to intracellular function - can also be disturbed by stress and other lifestyle factors;[158] whilst combining several stressful situations can have a synergistic and dramatic effect on their metabolism and can lead to the abolition of the circadian rhythm.[159]

	Thyroid Hormones
Thyroxine (T_4)	MAJOR product of the thyroid gland and the main thyroid hormone in the blood. It is a prohormone converted into either T_3 or rT_3 (mainly in the liver or kidneys).
Tri-iodothyronine (T_3)	Active and final form.

Reverse Tri-iodothyronine (rT$_3$)	Inactive form and major inhibitor of T$_3$ at cellular level. Can directly interfere with generation of T$_3$ from T$_4$.[160]

Increased cortisol levels produce a generalized pattern of lowered thyroid gland stimulation, and of decreased conversion to T$_3$ and increased conversion to rT$_3$.[161] Lifestyle, environmental and pathological events have also demonstrated this pattern - including stress, injury, illness, surgery, alcohol, calorie restriction, toxic metal exposure, diabetes mellitus and liver and kidney disease.[162] The effects of rT$_3$ are to slow metabolism and reduce cellular energy production (by blocking but not activating the receptors).[163] This generalized response may act as a protective feedback mechanism to prevent over-stimulation of the cells as a result of stress.

Such dysfunctional thyroid production has profound alterations on energy homeostasis at many levels, including glucose production and uptake, as well as fat breakdown; and has been linked with all components of the metabolic syndrome.[164] Because the liver has primary influence on the circulating levels of T$_3$ and rT$_3$, this organ plays a critical role in the production of active thyroid hormones.[165] Hence, supporting liver function is especially important. This links with the role of the liver in blood sugar control and the connection of blood sugar dysregulation and adrenal over-stimulation as underlying factors in thyroid hormone imbalances.

Mitochondrial Dysfunction

Mitochondria are the key organelles (specialised cellular structures) that play a central role in energy generation from nutrients[166] - they are your **cellular energy batteries**. Their numbers vary according to tissue type – from a singular organelle to several thousand.[167] Those tissues that require the most energy, such as muscles, will contain the largest numbers. In response to changes in energy demand and supply, the body adjusts both its *rate* (capacity) and/or *amount* (efficiency) of ATP production.[168] Dysfunction of these mitochondria plays a crucial role in metabolic disorders[169] and may be the underlying pathology of metabolic syndrome.[170]

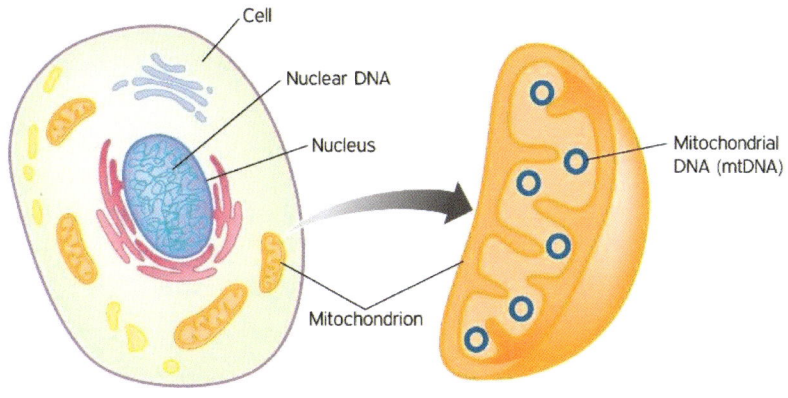

Source: www.imgsoup.com

In order to maintain healthy mitochondria, their structure changes continuously - switching between *fusion* (joining together) and *fission* (splitting of damaged material) in a sequentially repeating cycle.[171] These dynamics influence rate and amount, and provide a form of 'quality control' through elimination of damaged material.[172] Changes in their structure also provide a mechanism for adaption to metabolic demands and allows for a balance between energy demand and nutrient availability.[173] During feeding/nutrient excess (particularly high fat), fragmentation and high energy production rates can lead to damage and the excess generation of free radicals;[174] whereas during fasting/starvation, mitochondria tend to remain for longer in the connected state.[175] Disruption to the normal cycle can lead to abnormal function.[176]

Stress or cellular injury can shift the mitochondrial dynamics to fission resulting in mitochondrial fragmentation, which contributes to mitochondrial damage and consequent cell injury and cell death.[177] Pivotal in metabolic disorders are *oxidative stress* and inflammation.[178] Oxidative stress occurs mainly during ATP energy production and reflects an inability of the body's antioxidant mechanisms to fully counteract the free radicals generated through energy production. Left unchecked, these free radicals can cause extensive cellular damage and ATP depletion.[179] To prevent dysfunction within the mitochondria, it is necessary to support both antioxidant protection as well as nutrient-specific mitochondrial energy production.

Environmental Toxic Exposure

Environmental toxins are now also being causally linked to the metabolic syndrome,[180] especially chemical toxins that can disrupt hormone function and impact on mitochondrial function. The Stockholm Convention identified a range of pesticides, industrial chemicals and their by-products that caused such disruption.[181] These were termed **POPs (persistent organic pollutants)** and defined as *"chemical substances that persist in the environment, bio-accumulate through the food web, and pose a risk of causing adverse effects to human health and the environment"*. An association has subsequently been confirmed between serum POPs (which accumulate over years) and the metabolic syndrome.[182]

Other major causes of cellular toxicity include **heavy metals**, which are natural components of the Earth's crust and are the oldest toxins known to humans. Virtually all heavy metals are toxic in sufficient quantities. However, those that have the most serious health implications are arsenic, lead, cadmium and mercury[183] - all of which are ubiquitous air and water pollutants.[184]

Sources of Heavy Metal Toxicity[185][186]	
Natural sources (e.g. groundwater, metal ores)	Industrial processes
Commercial products (e.g. cleaning products)	Contaminated food (especially large fish)
Occupational exposure	Air pollution
Smoking	Stainless steel saucepans
Dental amalgam	

Heavy metals produce toxicity by forming complexes with cellular compounds, which inactivate enzyme systems or modify critical structures through oxidative stress inducement.[187] This can lead to cellular dysfunction, impairment in mitochondrial ATP production, energy depletion, and cellular death.[188] The generation of oxidative stress is considered one of the major mechanisms behind heavy metal toxicity;[189] whilst chemical toxicity – both heavy metal and other chemical toxins – is now being linked with mitochondrial dysfunction and the pathogenesis of CFS/ME.[190] Hence, it may be necessary to support antioxidant and detoxification pathways; and in the case of heavy metal accumulation, to consider using **chelators** - charged molecules that can bind to heavy metals to form a neutral complex which can be excreted by the kidney.[191]

PART TWO:
The Energy Programme Plan

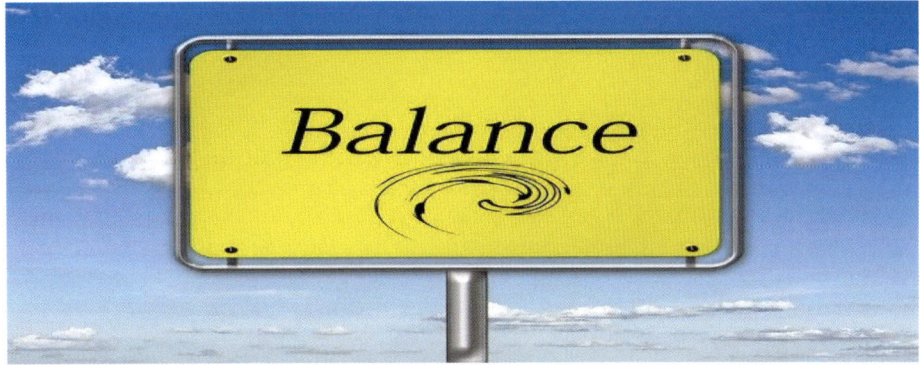

Source: www.pixabay.com

Overview

The key to any health improvement programme is to develop a life-long plan that makes you feel great, gives you more energy, balances your mood and reduces your risk of disease. It is not about strict dietary limitations, depriving yourself of foods and other things that you love or even staying unrealistically thin. This programme plan is designed as a series of progressive steps for you to implement within your own timeframe. It is very much in recognition of the fact that we all find change difficult and that trying to introduce too much change at once will inevitably result in failure as we become overwhelmed. Remember that every change that you make counts, no matter how small and even if you temporarily relapse to your old ways. Do not let any relapses derail you though. Simply revert back to the plan and know that you have already started on your journey to the sustained energy that you desire.

The Programme Plan			
1.	Hydration	5.	Supplements
2.	Sleep	6.	Exercise
3.	Stress Management	7.	Stimulants
4.	Diet		

Chapter 7: Hydration

The Starting Point

The KEY starting point in this plan is effective hydration. Most of us are simply not sufficiently hydrated enough, which manifests in tiredness or hunger. Proper hydration, however, requires more than water alone. It also requires certain minerals, called **electrolytes,** which help regulate fluid balance within the body. Water, though, is the number one priority.

Water Requirements

The amount of water required per day varies from individual to individual and will depend upon various factors, including the type of environment, how much energy is exerted during the day and whether you are male or female. In general, *the amount required per day by the average sedentary adult is:* [192]

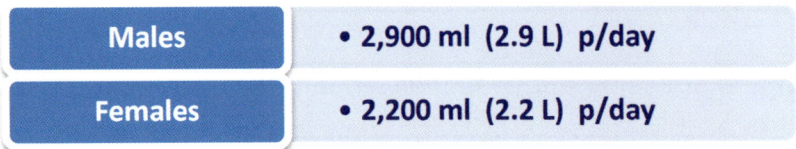

These amounts generally come from solid foods, which contribute approximately 1 L, with the remainder coming from decaffeinated and non-alcoholic drinks.[193] Caffeinated drinks are not as effective as they can exert a minor diuretic effect (although less so than was previously thought).[194] However, if you are exposed to a hot environment or physical exercise, then you will require more fluids because you will have increased water loss through sweating. Runners, for example, can lose in their sweat between *1.0-2.5 L/hr of fluid* (or more in hot environments). Be aware also, that water is lost daily through the production of urine, faeces and the breath, so regular replenishment is necessary.

The Electrolytes

Electrolytes are a group of minerals that carry an electrical charge when dissolved in water. They are essential to proper fluid balance within the body by regulating fluid passage across cell membranes. Cells need to be bathed in fluids, both inside and out, in order to function properly. However, too much fluid inside of the cells will cause them to become water-logged and impair their function, so fluids need to be kept in balance between the inside and outside of the cells.

Fluid regulation occurs through a process called *osmosis*, whereby water in the body moves into regions with a higher solute concentration to dilute that concentration - i.e. water follows the charged minerals, which are the solutes (substances dissolved in water).

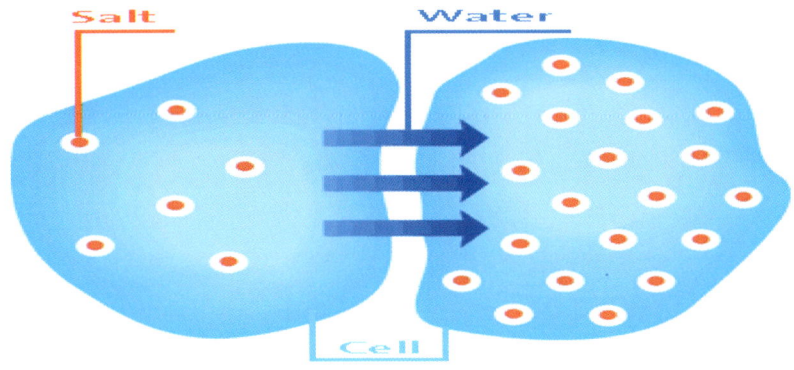

Source: www.pixshark.com

Sodium is the main electrolyte found outside of the cells, whilst **potassium** is the main electrolyte found inside of the cells. The most common electrolyte imbalances are in sodium and potassium. Often too much sodium is consumed in the form of processed foods, which are high in salt, whilst too little potassium is consumed through a lack of intake of fruits and vegetables, leading to an imbalance between the two minerals. Disturbances in their levels can cause fatigue and, in extreme cases, can lead to cardiac and neurological complications, which may result in a medical emergency.

Conversely, sodium levels can become dangerously depleted through sweat loss in hot environments and/or through exercise. Exercise-associated **hyponatremia** (low blood sodium levels) has emerged as the most common life-threatening complication of endurance exercise.[195] In such cases, sweat-induced sodium loss leads to sodium depletion, excessive water loss and dehydration. Without sodium, the body is unable to hold on to water. Consequently, one of the main functions of the kidneys is to reabsorb sodium and prevent sodium being lost in the urine.

When there is such sodium depletion, a condition of *over-hydration* can then occur if too much water is then consumed without replacing the lost sodium. In this situation, the decrease in the sodium concentration outside of the cells lowers the fluid osmotic pressure and results in too much water flowing into the cells and effectively water-logging the cells. This severe over-hydration is known as *water intoxication* and is especially problematic for marathon runners who have lost a lot of sweat during the race and have then tried to replace their water loss with water alone. Consequences of such water intoxication can also be serious and fatal.

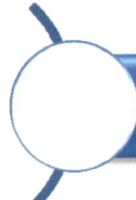

Effective hydration = water + sodium

Quick Reference Dehydration Chart

This simple chart is an easy-to-use tool for you to check your hydration levels. It is based on the colour of your urine. **The darker the colour, the greater is your dehydration.**

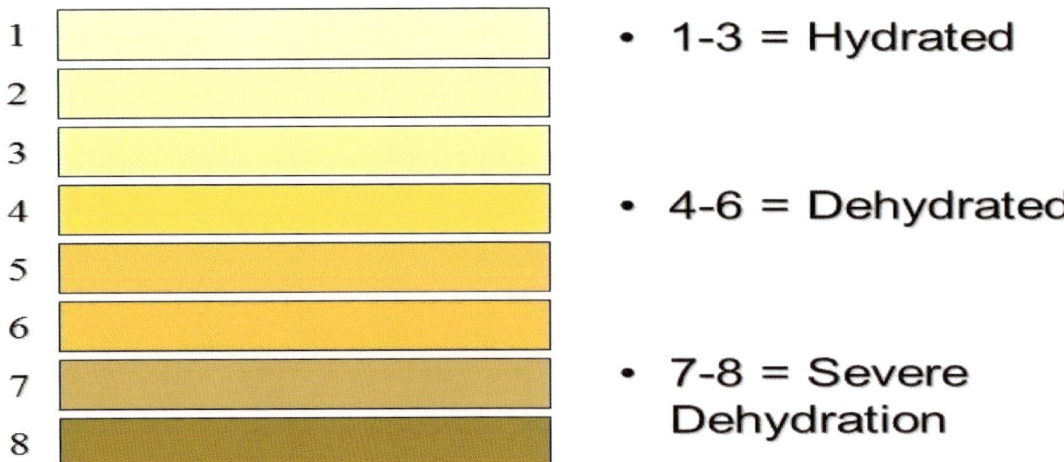

Be Aware! If you are taking a vitamin or a multi-vitamin and mineral supplement, some of the vitamins in the supplement can change the colour of your urine for a few hours, making it bright yellow or discoloured.

Key Action Points

Daily Intake	• Aim to drink approx. 1.5 L of water &/or non-caffeinated drinks throughout the day
Thirst	• Do NOT ignore - you are alredy dehydrated
Heat	• Increase your water intake in hot environments
Sweat	• Increase your water and sodium (salt) intake
Exercise	• Consume both water and salt after exercise
Caffeine	• Reduce/eliminate caffeinated drinks

Chapter 8: Sleep

Sleep Deprivation

Sleep has a direct impact on your daytime functioning and your energy levels. It is generally accepted that it serves to permit recovery from previous wakefulness and/or prepares for functioning in the subsequent wake period. However, such is the current scale of sleep deprivation that the *Centres for Disease Control and Prevention* in the US has declared that insufficient sleep is now a public health epidemic, with an estimated 50-70 million US adults having a sleep or wakefulness disorder.[196] In the UK, the figure is around 1 in 3 adults.[197]

Biological Function

Physiological processes, learning, memory and cognition are all significantly affected by sleep.[198] Restricting sleep to less than 6 hours per night can impair cognitive performance and mood,[199] glucose metabolism,[200] appetite regulation,[201] and immune function.[202] All of which can have a significant impact on metabolism. This corresponds with a greater likelihood of metabolic disorders such as obesity, diabetes and hypertension in those suffering with sleep insufficiency.[203] Such evidence is the basis for the recommendation that adults should obtain 8 hours of sleep per night.[204]

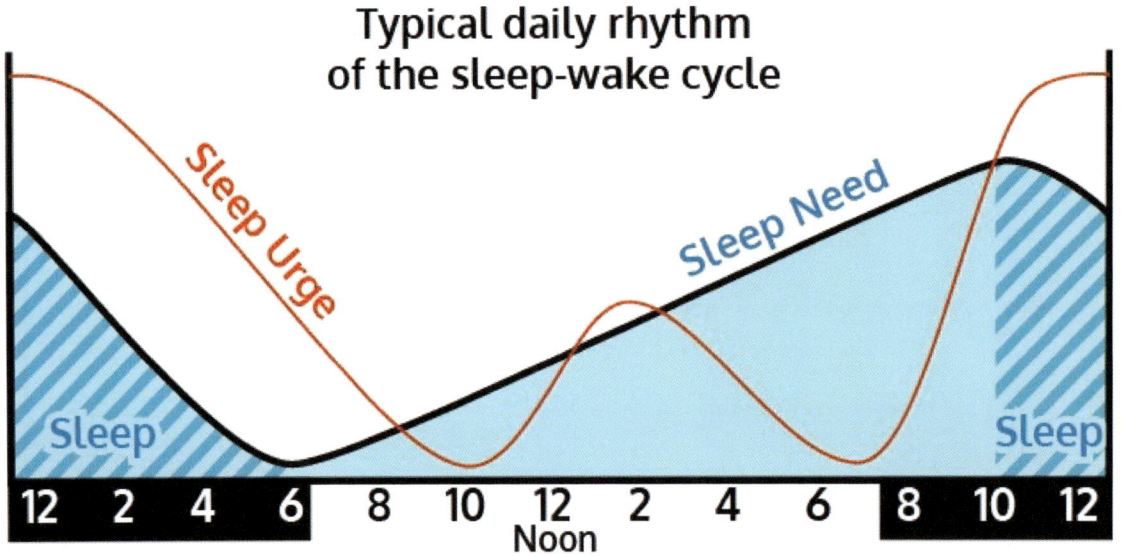

Source: www.waterpoloplanet.com

The Sleep-Wake Cycle

The sleep-wake cycle is governed by the primary circadian clock - the *suprachiasmatic nucleus (SCN)* of the hypothalamus - via the action of light on the eyes providing information as to whether it is day or night. In response to darkness, the hormone *melatonin* (which promotes sleep) is produced from the pineal gland in the brain. Secretion peaks at night and ebbs during the day. Its rhythm contrasts with that of cortisol (the hormone that gets you up in the morning and keeps you awake and active), which peaks in the morning and ebbs in the evening. Both melatonin and cortisol secretion rhythms are directly regulated by the SCN and act as the major hormonal pathways that communicate with the SCN.[205] Together, these two hormones stabilise the circadian rhythm.[206]

The only external stimuli that affects melatonin synthesis is retinal light exposure.[207] However, cortisol production is influenced by several interacting systems, not just the master clock.[208] Being highly stress-responsive, cortisol's natural rhythm can be disrupted by external factors, such as sleep-restriction, day-time sleeping, jetlag,[209] changes in lighting, feeding schedules and physical activity.[210] These can lead to high cortisol levels in the evening, which in turn can lower or delay melatonin production because melatonin onset typically occurs during low cortisol secretion.[211] Such disruption to these two main clock regulatory hormones can lead to 'out-of-synch' rhythms in biological processes, resulting in an array of symptoms.[212] Although stressors need to be addressed, **the key factor in re-setting the biological clock is *light***, as this can advance or delay the circadian rhythm, thereby directly impacting health.[213]

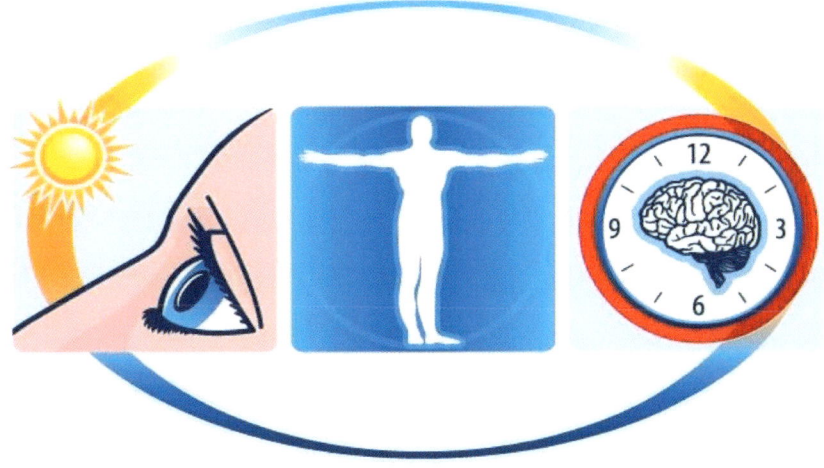

Source: www.lightingforhealth.com

Jetlag and Shift Work

Jetlag and sleep disturbances (such as sleep restriction or shift work) result in a transient mismatch between the internal circadian time and the external light-dark cycle.[214] Symptoms of jetlag include decreased alertness, motor coordination and cognitive performance; as well as sleep disturbances, gastrointestinal disruption and loss of appetite.[215] Sleep restriction and daytime sleep (hallmarks of night shift work) are associated with increased BMI (body mass index), risk of the metabolic syndrome and alterations in cortisol, insulin and glucose.[216] In both cases, cortisol rhythms are affected - even where only three or fewer time zones are crossed by plane[217] or where there are relatively subtle advances in sleep timing.[218]

It is the abruptness of the changes in both cases that causes the problems as the circadian timing system cannot adapt so quickly to the new time schedule.[219] Jetlag is also often exacerbated by the effects of sleep loss, which usually accompanies long-distance travel;[220] whilst flying eastwards is more taxing on the body because the internal clock has to be re-set earlier; and travelling across multiple time zones increases the severity and length of symptoms as it takes longer to re-set the circadian pacemaker.[221] For most of us, jetlag is self-resolving but for those who travel frequently for work, short-term health problems can ensure;[222] whereas for airline flight crews there can be long-term health consequences.[223]

Problems associated with shift-work are more widespread. In the US, many of the estimated 9% of Americans (12.5 million) who work on the night shift or on irregular rotating/shift schedules overnight experience sleep and health disorders.[224] In the UK, the percentage of the population working shifts is even higher at 14%,[225] which equates to approximately 9 million people. This means that a staggering number of people are affected by circadian clock disruptions that lead to a significantly increased risk of metabolic disorders such as energy disruption, obesity, diabetes and hypertension.[226]

Sleep Hygiene

Sleep hygiene is the name given to the promotion of good sleep habits and regular sleep. Well planned strategies are essential to promote long-term deep, restorative sleep. However, everyone is different – what works for one person may not work for another. Although most of us require around eight hours of sleep each night, sleep requirements do vary from person to person. So, you need to determine in the first instance how much sleep is enough for you – that's the amount of time you need to sleep in order to wake up feeling refreshed and rejuvenated. There are a number of techniques that you can use to help promote good sleep but the key is to experiment with those techniques to find what works best for you.

General Sleeping Tips[227]

The starting point is to **discover your optimal sleep schedule**. Experiment with different sleep and wake times. Go to bed at the same time every night and allow yourself to wake up naturally. If you are sleep deprived, it may take a few weeks to fully recover. Eventually you will find the sleep schedule that works for you. Once you have discovered your optimal sleep times, then the following tips will help you to regulate your sleep to ensure that you get the deep, restorative sleep that you need.

Tip 1 - Keep a regular sleep schedule	
Set a regular bedtime	Go to bed at the same time every night at a time when you normally feed tired. Try not to break this routine on weekends.
Wake up at the same time every day	If you are getting enough sleep, you should wake up naturally without an alarm. Otherwise, set an earlier bedtime.
Nap to make up for lost sleep	Take a nap for less than 30 mins to make up for lost sleep rather than sleeping late to prevent sleep-wake rhythm disruption.
Fight after-dinner drowsiness	If you get sleepy before bedtime, do something mildly stimulating, such as washing the dishes or calling a friend.

Tip 2 - Naturally regulate your sleep-wake cycle	
Increase light exposure during the day	Use work breaks and exercise to spend more time outside. Keep curtains/blinds open or use a light therapy box if you are exposed to very little natural daylight in your office.

Boost melatonin production at night	Avoid bright lights before bed. Turn off your TV or computer and don't read from a back-lit device (such as an iPad). Make sure the room is dark when it is time to sleep or use a sleep mask.

Tip 3 - Create a relaxing bedtime routine	
Make your bedroom more sleep friendly	Sleep on a comfortable mattress and pillow and have enough room to stretch and turn. Keep the room cool and ventilated. Use ear plugs, soothing sounds or white noise to reduce noise.
Reserve your bed for sleeping and sex	Use your bed only for sleep or sex to provide cues for sleep or romance. Avoid doing work or other things in bed.
Try some relaxing bedtime rituals	Read by a soft light. Take a warm bath. Listen to soft music or audio books. Do some easy stretches. Prepare for the next day.

Tip 4 – Eat right and get regular exercise	
Watch what you consume in the hours before bed	Avoid big/heavy meals within 2 hours of bed. Eat a light snack if hungry. Avoid alcohol and smoking as they are both stimulants that reduce your sleep quality and will wake you up in the night.
Exercise daily	Include 20-30 minutes of activity such as housework, gardening or walking. Break the time into smaller chunks throughout the day if pushed for time. Use gentle exercise in the evening.

Tip 5 – Keep anxiety and stress in check	
Learn how to manage your thoughts	Employ stress management techniques to reduce stress, remain calm and manage your time effectively. *See Chapter 9.*
Employ relaxation techniques	Try deep breathing, progressive muscle relaxation, visualization and meditation. CDs can guide you through the techniques.

Tip 6 – Ways to get back to sleep	
Stay out of your head	Remain in bed in a relaxed position without focusing on your wakefulness. Instead, focus on feelings/sensations in your body.
Make relaxation your goal and not sleep	Try one of the relaxation techniques above. Remind yourself that rest and relaxation still help to rejuvenate your body.
Do non-stimulating activity after 30 minutes	Get out of bed and read without a back-lit device. Keep the lights dim. Eat a light snack to raise your blood sugar.
Postpone worrying	Make a brief note of anything making your feel anxious. Deal with it the next day when it will be easier to resolve.

Tip 7 – Cope with shift-work sleep disorder	
Limit the consecutive number of shifts	If that is not possible, avoid rotating shifts frequently so that you can maintain the same sleep schedule.
Avoid a long commute	This will increase sleep time and limit the time spent travelling home in daylight.
Drink caffeinated drinks early in your shift.	This will stimulate your energy for your work but avoid close to your bedtime as caffeine will keep you awake.
Take frequent breaks	Use the breaks to move around as much as possible. Take a walk, stretch or exercise if possible.
Adjust your sleep-wake schedule	Use bright lights when you wake up and bright lamps/bulbs in your workplace. Wear dark glasses on your way home.
Eliminate noise and light from your bedroom	Use blackout curtains /sleep mask and ear plugs/soothing sounds to block out daytime light/noise. Turn off your phone.
Make sleep a priority at the weekends	Or on your non-working days so you can pay off your sleep debt.

Tip 8 – Know when to see a doctor	
See a doctor if the tips have not helped and you have the following symptoms:	<ul><li>Persistent daytime sleepiness or fatigue</li><li>Loud snoring accompanied by pauses in breathing</li><li>Difficulty falling asleep or staying asleep</li><li>Unrefreshing sleep</li><li>Frequent morning headaches</li><li>Crawling sensations in your legs or arms at night</li><li>Inability to move while falling asleep or waking up</li><li>Physically acting out dreams during sleep</li><li>Falling asleep at inappropriate times</li></ul>

Chapter 9: Stress Management

Stress Response

Stress is a major contributor to energy disruption. The stress mechanism will respond to any challenge that the body faces, whether real or perceived, and to do that it requires energy. ***However:***

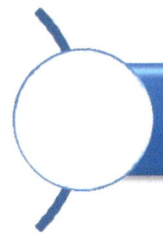

It is YOUR response to stress rather than the size of the actual stress that is important.

Hence, you have more control over the stress in your life than you think. The simple realisation that you are in control of your life is the foundation of stress management. **Managing stress is all about taking charge of your thoughts, emotions, schedule and the way that you deal with problems.**

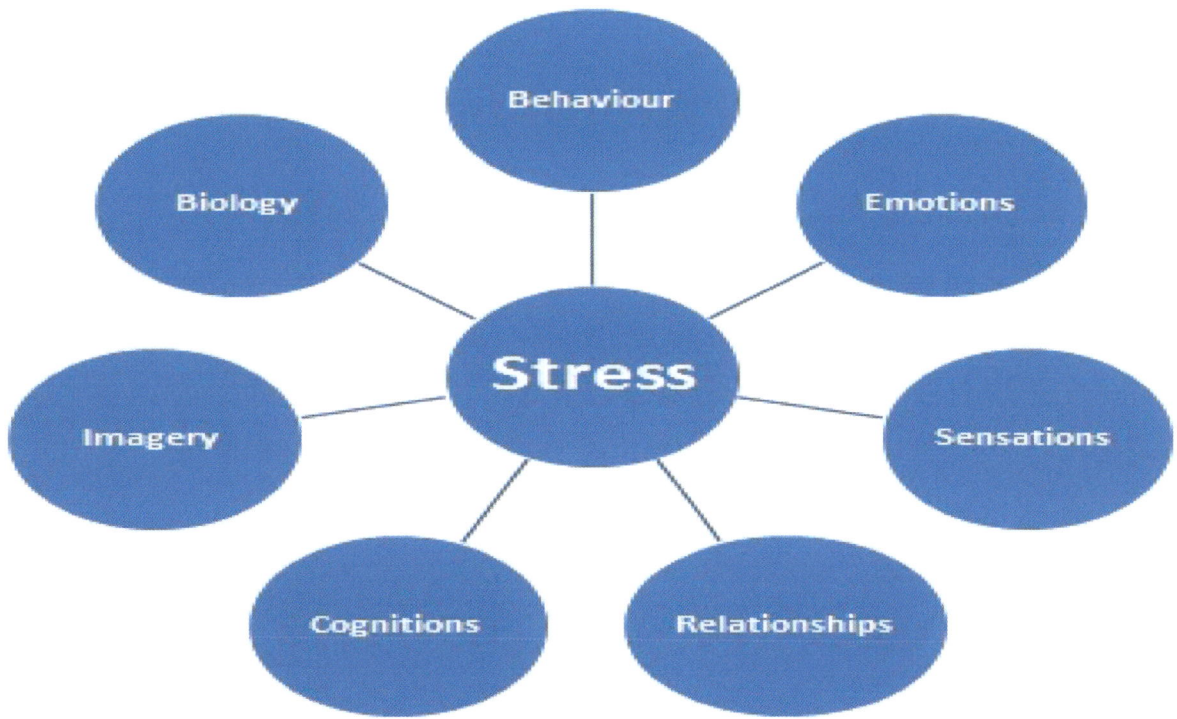

There are a number of strategies that you can adopt to help you cope with stress but the starting point is always to identify the source(s) of your stress.

Stress Source Identification

This is not as easy as it sounds as your true stress sources are not always obvious. It is easy to blame work demands, outside events or other people, especially when you are juggling multiple demands. However, what are often over-looked are your own stress-inducing thoughts, feelings and behaviours that lead to the stress. For example, it may be that it is your procrastination rather than the actual job demands that lead to deadline stress. To identify your stress sources you need to look closely at your own habits, attitudes and excuses. Until you accept responsibility for the role you play in creating or maintaining stress, your level will remain outside of your control.

Stress Journal

Starting a **Stress Journal** can help you to identify the regular stressors in your life and the way that you deal with them. Keep a daily log of how you are feeling. Log all of your stressful events. Include what caused or what your think caused your stress; how you felt, both physically and emotionally; and how you acted in response. You will soon begin to see patterns and common themes. Once you have established the patterns and themes, you will then be in a position to start addressing them and to take back control of your life.

Stress Coping Methods

There are many healthy ways to manage and cope with stress, just as there are many unhealthy strategies that many people employ that temporarily reduce stress but cause more damage in the long run. By examining your stress coping methods, you can learn to recognise and eliminate the unhealthy strategies and replace them with healthy ones. Unhealthy strategies include:

Unhealthy Coping Strategies		
Smoking	Drinking too much	Overeating/under-eating
Watching too much TV	Excessive computer use	Sleeping too much
Procrastinating	Social withdrawal	Lashing out at others

Healthy coping strategies require CHANGE.
You can either change the SITUATION or change your REACTION.

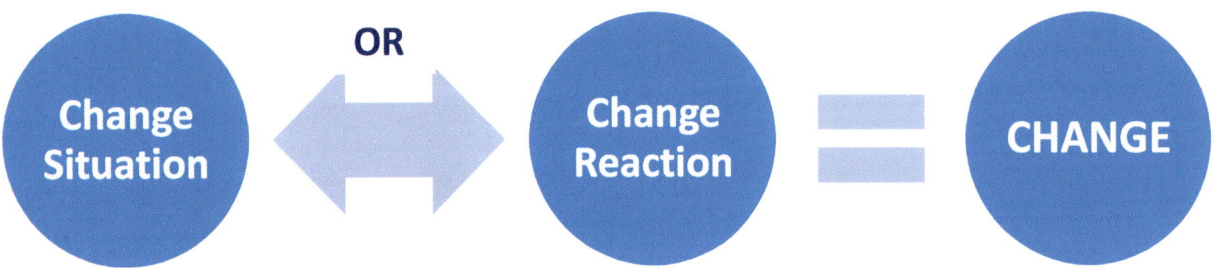

Change Instigation

If you choose to change the situation you can either *avoid or alter* the stressor; whereas if you choose to change your reaction you can either *adapt or accept* the stressor. No single method works for everyone or in every situation, so experiment with different techniques and strategies and focus on what makes you feel calm and in control. When choosing your options, consider the *four As*: *avoid, alter, adapt or accept*.

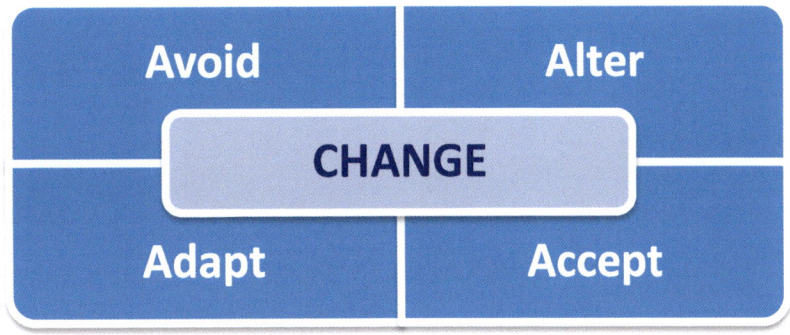

To avoid becoming overwhelmed or 'stressed' by the prospect of stress control, start small. Pick one problem and try the strategies listed below to see if they work for you.

Stress Management Strategies[228]

Strategy 1 – Avoid unnecessary stress	
Not all stress can be avoided and it is not healthy to avoid a situation that needs to be addressed. However, many stressors can be safely eliminated.	
Learn to say "NO"	Know your limits and don't take on more than you can handle.

Avoid stressful people	End the relationship or limit your time with them.
Control your environment	Change your routine, even if you have to go out of your way.
Avoid hot-button topics	Cross contentious issues off your conversation list.
Reduce your 'to-do' list	Relegate non-urgent tasks or eliminate entirely.

Strategy 2 – Alter the situation

If you can't avoid the situation, change what you can do to prevent it in the future. Often, this involves changing the way that you communicate.

Express your feelings	Not bottling up your feelings will prevent resentment building.
Willingness to compromise	Change your behavior as well as asking others to change theirs.
Be more assertive	Deal with problems head on to prevent re-occurrence.
Manage your time	Plan ahead and don't over-extend yourself.

Strategy 3 – Adapt to the stressor

If you can't change the stressor, change yourself. By changing your expectations and attitudes you can adapt to the stressor and regain your sense of control.

Reframe problems	View stressful situations from a more positive perspective.
Look at the big picture	Put the stress into the long-term perspective.
Adjust your standards	Set reasonable standards for you and others and not perfection.
Focus on the positive	Learn to appreciate all the good and positive in your life.
Adjust your attitude	Replace self-defeating thoughts with positive thoughts.

Strategy 4 – Accept the things that you cannot change

Some sources of stress are unavoidable. In such cases, the best way to cope is to accept things as they are. It is easier than railing against a situation that you cannot change.

Refocus the uncontrollable	Focus on what you can control such as your reaction.
Look for the upside	Look at challenges as opportunities for personal growth.

Share your feelings	With a friend or therapist. It can be very cathartic.
Learn to forgive	Let go of anger and resentments to release negative energy.

Strategy 5 – Adopt a healthy lifestyle

You can increase your resistance to stress and improve your ability to cope by strengthening your physical health.

Eat a healthy diet	Provides the nutrients for the stress response function.
Exercise regularly	Physical activity can reduce and prevent stress effects.
Reduce caffeine and sugar	To prevent mood and energy swings from blood sugar lows.
Avoid alcohol and smoking	Deal with the problem head on rather than avoiding the issue.
Get enough sleep	A rejuvenated body can copy better with stress.

Strategy 6 – Make time for fun and relaxation

Nurturing yourself is an effective way to reduce stress. It is a necessity not a luxury. If you regularly make time for fun and relaxation, you will be better able to handle stressors.

Set aside relaxation time	Include every day and don't allow other obligations to encroach.
Connect with others	Spend time with positive people who enhance your life.
Do something you enjoy	Every day make time for leisure activities that bring you joy.
Keep your humour	Including your ability to laugh at yourself.
Find healthy ways to relax and recharge	

Go for a walk	Play with a pet
Spend time in nature	Listen to music
Call a good friend	Watch a comedy
Sweat out tension with exercise	Get a massage
Write in a journal	Read a good book
Take a long bath	Laugh
Light scented candles	Work in your garden

Chapter 10: Diet

The Goal

Healthy eating is about developing a life-long eating plan that makes you feel great, gives you more energy, balances your mood and reduces your risk of disease. It is not about strict dietary limitations, depriving yourself of foods that you love or staying unrealistically thin. **Key aspects are moderation and balance.** Moderation means eating only as much food as your body needs, so that you feel satisfied at the end of a meal but not stuffed. Whereas balance refers to the need to include a good balance of foods from all the major food groups - carbohydrates, proteins, fats, vitamins, minerals and phytonutrients.

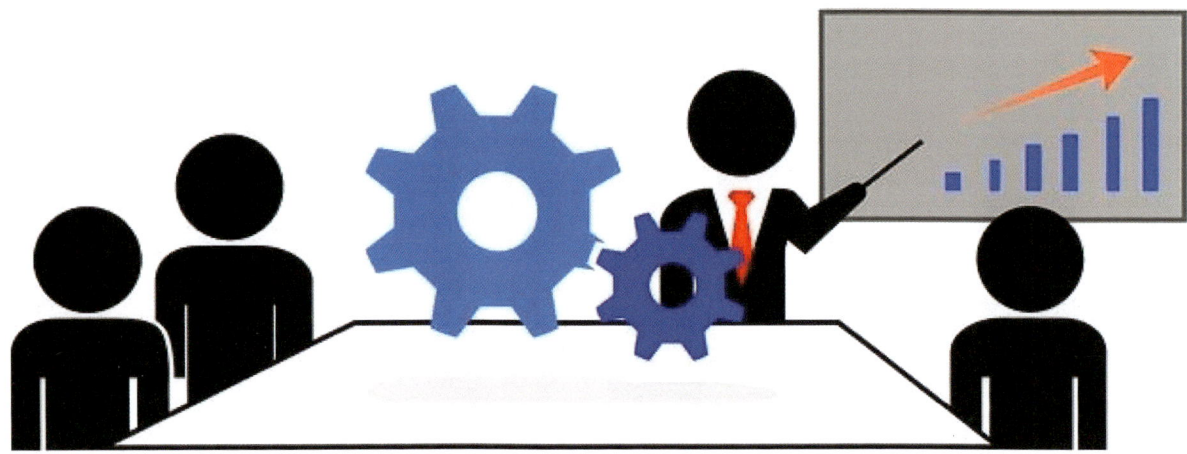

Source: www.pixaby.com

Learn the Basics	
No Limits	Do not try to eliminate completely certain foods, even unhealthy ones. You will only start to crave them.
Reduce Unhealthy Choices	Reduce the number of times that you eat junk food to lessen their impact. Your cravings will also start to reduce.
Reduce Portion Size	Reduce portion size by using smaller plates. Such visual cues can help your brain control portion size.
Learn Balance	If you do blow out on unhealthy food, then simply balance it out at the next meal with healthy choices.

Set Yourself up for Success

Plan a healthy diet as a number of small, manageable steps rather than one big drastic change and learn to re-connect with your food. How you *think* about food is just as important as what you are eating. Taking the time to slow down and think about the food that you are eating as nourishment will allow time for the body's satiety signals to kick in and will bring back the enjoyment of eating. Gulping down food to just fill a hole in your stomach will lead to mindless overeating. If you approach the changes gradually and with commitment, you will have a healthy diet sooner than you think.

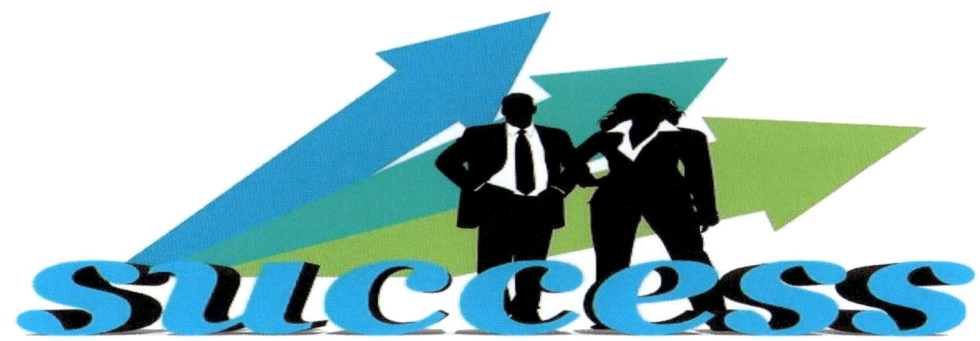

Source: www.pixabay.com

Get Your Mind-Set Right	
Simplify	Think in terms of colour, variety and freshness and focus on finding foods that you love.
Start Slowly	Make small changes to your diet. As these become habit, continue to add more healthy choices.
Change Matters	Every change made counts, even if you relapse to your old ways. Don't let hiccups derail you.
Drink Water	Ensure you are well hydrated to prevent tiredness. Thirst signals can often be mistaken for hunger signals. Try drinking water when you feel hungry.
Eat Regularly	Do not skip meals and eat small snacks during the day to prevent cravings and provide sustained energy.
Eat with Others	Allows you to model healthy eating habits and has numerous social and emotional benefits.

Eat Slowly	Take time to chew your food and taste the flavours and textures. Learn to enjoy eating again.
Stop Eating Early	Stop eating before you feel full. It takes a few minutes for your brain to tell your body that it has had enough.

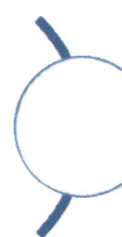

KNOW THE FOOD GROUPS

Carbohydrates

Carbohydrates are the main fuel of the body and provide the energy for you to function. They are made up of chains of sugar units that are linked together and are broken down to a single sugar unit. The length of the chain determines the speed at which the molecule is digested. The more complex the chain, the longer it takes to digest and the better it is at keeping you full longer and providing sustained energy. The shorter the chain, the quicker the molecule is digested and the greater you will experience energy fluctuations, cravings and mood swings. Hence, complex carbohydrates are the *"good carbs"*.

Source: www.pixabay.com

Carbohydrates include whole grains, beans, vegetables and fruits. The refined versions, however, have had their nutrients and fibre removed during processing and should be avoided as they can lead to widely fluctuating energy, moods and sugar cravings. These include white grains, such as white bread, pasta, rice and pastries, as well as the likes of biscuits, cakes and pies – anything that has been processed essentially. These are the *"bad carbs"*.

Complex Carbs (unrefined)	Refined Carbs
Wholegrain cereals – wheat, rice, oats, barley, rye, millet, buckwheat, quinoa	White cereals – white wheat, rice, pearl barley, non-wholegrain oats
Wholegrain bread, pasta, noodles	White bread, pasta, noodles
Beans, peas, legumes, lentils	Commercial breakfast cereals
Vegetables and fruit	Pastries, cakes, biscuits, sweets, chocolate
Honey (some)	Crisps, pizza, chips, fizzy drinks, sugar, jam

KEY components of any healthy eating programme are fruit and vegetables. They are low in calories and nutrient dense; which means they are packed with vitamins, minerals, phytonutrients, antioxidants and fibre. Each colour provides different benefits, whilst the deeper and richer the colour, the higher is the concentration of nutrients. Along with other complex carbohydrates, they are also high in fibre which is vital to gut health. There are two types of fibre: soluble and insoluble. *Soluble fibres* attract water and form a gel, which slows down digestion and absorption. This can help you feel full and provide a sustained energy release. Conversely, *insoluble fibres* do not dissolve in water; so they pass through the GI tract relatively intact and speed up the passage of food and waste through your gut, which helps gut motility and can prevent constipation.

Soluble Fibre	Insoluble Fibre
Oats	Mainly wholegrains and vegetables
Lentils, beans, peas, nuts	Wheat, barley, rice, couscous, bulgar wheat, corn, rye
Flaxseeds, psyllium	Nuts, seeds
Cucumber, celery, carrots	Fruit, grapes, raisins
Apples, oranges, pears, strawberries, blueberries	Celery, broccoli, cabbage, onions, tomatoes, carrots, courgettes, green beans, dark green leafy vegetables, root vegetable skins

Insoluble fibres are considered *gut-healthy* because they feed the *"good bacteria"* of the gut and are hence termed **prebiotics**. Gut microbiota produce short-chain fatty acids (SCFAs), such as butyrate, from bacterial fermentation of insoluble fibre.[229] The increased gut concentration of butyrate is associated with an improvement in metabolic health.[230] Positive metabolic health effects include satiety increase, lower cholesterol levels and glucose regulation.[231] SCFAs also trigger cellular signalling cascades that modulate inflammation and control body energy utilisation.[232] A lack of butyrate appears to play an important role in the pathology of obesity; hence a fibre enriched diet can help to protect against obesity and insulin resistance.[233]

Manage Your Carbs	
Eat Healthy Carbs	At each meal, eat some form of healthy carbohydrate: whole grains, beans/legumes, vegetables and fruits.
Avoid Unhealthy Carbs	Avoid the white refined foods such as breads, pastas, rice, breakfast cereals, pastries, cakes, biscuits and sugar.
White to Brown	Start switching your white grains to their brown whole grain equivalents. Mix the types at first if necessary.
Variety	Introduce a variety of whole grains, including whole wheat, brown rice, millet, quinoa, barley, oats and rye.
100% Whole Grain	Some brown grains are only partial whole grains. Look for the words "whole grain" on the ingredients list.
Rainbow Colours	Eat a variety of different coloured fruit and vegetables each day. The brighter the colour the better.
5 Portions of Fruit & Vegetable per day	Aim for a minimum of five portions of fruit and vegetables each day. The greater the number and variety, the greater the benefits.
Include Insoluble Fibre	Make sure that each day you eat some food that includes insoluble fibre.

Fats

Fats are just as important to your diet as other types of nutrients. Over the years they have had a bad press and have been linked to multiple health problems from obesity to high cholesterol and cardiovascular disease. The message has been to avoid fats if you want to be healthy. But this misses the point that fats are essential to your health. ***The key is to differentiate between the good and the bad fats.*** The omega-3 and omega-6 unsaturated fats are absolutely essential because they cannot be made by the body and must be eaten regularly in the diet. They have multiple functions, including hormonal and structural properties. Even cholesterol is essential. Cholesterol is the raw material from which all of your steroid hormones are made. They include the hormones that govern your stress response, your metabolism and even your sexual hormone cycle. Such is the importance of cholesterol, that the body makes its own!

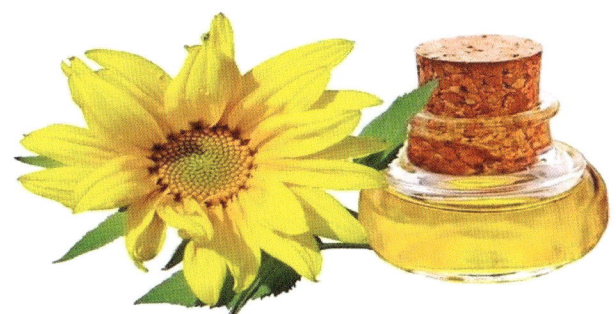

Source: www.pixabay.com

The fats to avoid are the trans-fats. These are fats that have been altered chemically through processing, usually through hydrogenation. The fats may start off as healthy by using omega-6 oils, such as sunflower oil. But once altered, these fats can cause disruption to bodily processes by blocking enzyme systems, which can ultimately lead to health problems. Margarine is a classic example of a healthy omega-6 fat that is turned into an unhealthy trans-fat. Revert back to butter, it's much healthier.

Saturated Fats	Omega-3 Unsaturated	Omega-6 Unsaturated
Meat (including processed meat such as sausages & bacon)	Oily fish (tuna, salmon, mackerel, sardines, herring, trout)	Oils of safflower, sunflower, sesame, pumpkin
Fish	Linseeds (AKA flaxseeds)	Walnut oil
Dairy – cheese, butter, milk	Hempseed	Borage oil
Chocolate	Soya bean	Evening primrose oil
Coconut, palm oil, lard	Algal oil	Meat & animal products

Over the past century, there has been a significant decrease in omega-3 fatty acid intake and a relative increase in omega-6 fatty acids, leading to an increase in the omega-6/omega-3 ratio from 2:1 to about 16:1.[234] These two essential fats need to be kept in balance because of their opposing effects; otherwise health consequences can ensue, including energy dysregulation. Hence, it is important to restore the correct ratio balance between these essential fats.

	Re-Balance Your Fats
Increase Omega-3 Fats	Aim to eat 3 portions of oily fish per week, such as: salmon, tuna, mackerel, sardines, anchovies. Regularly eat seeds/nuts or their oils high in omega-3, such as flaxseeds, chia seeds and walnuts.
Decrease Omega-6 Fats	Substitute your use of cooking oils such as sunflower/safflower oil with olive oil - which is low in omega-6 but relatively stable for cooking at low temperature - or coconut oil for high temperatures. Obtain your omega-6 fats from lean and fresh meat and other animal products. If vegetarian, include oils such as borage oil and pumpkin seeds.
Avoid/Restrict Trans-Fats	Avoid or restrict intake of margarines, crackers, biscuits, sweets, snack foods, fried foods, baked goods, and other processed foods.

Proteins

Proteins are crucial to virtually every process within your body. They are the building blocks of body tissue but they can also serve as a fuel source. They are essential for maintaining cells, tissues and organs; and form the basis of your enzymes, hormones and immune cells. Without protein, your body would cease to function. Nutritionally, the most important aspect of protein is the composition of its amino acids (basic protein units). There are 20 amino acids, of which nine are essential and so must be taken in via the diet as the body cannot make them. These essential amino acids need to be in a certain ratio, which gives rise to a type of ranking system for protein sources. Animal proteins contain the correct ratios and so are considered 'complete'; whereas vegetable protein sources do not and so are considered 'incomplete'. Vegetarians and vegans must eat a variety of plant sources to obtain the complete ratios.

High Quality	Medium Quality	Poor Quality
Meat	Beans, legumes, soya, peas	Other seeds
Fish	Pumpkin, hemp, chia seeds	Grains (except buckwheat)
Fowl	Nuts	Vegetables
Eggs and dairy	Spirulina	Fruits

Protein is the most satiating macronutrient,[235] as it stimulates the release of the hormone cholecystokinin (CCK) in the gut, which reduces food intake and induces satiety.[236] In general, increased satiety occurs after meals with a protein content of ≥ 25%.[237] Increased satiety helps to decrease energy intake and increase energy expenditure through an increased thermic effect (heat production).[238] High protein diets have been shown to prevent the development of diet-induced obesity and, in animal studies, improve metabolic disorders.[239]

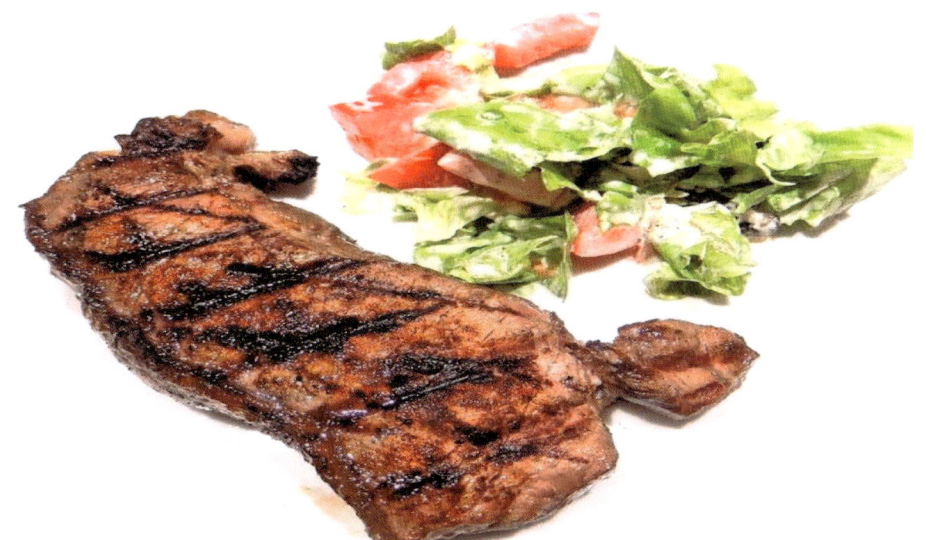

Source: www.pixabay.com

Most people simply do not get enough protein to power the numerous bodily functions on a daily basis, let alone during times of stress when the requirement for protein increases. Eating protein at each meal and with each snack will ensure an adequate supply and will help to balance your energy levels through a more sustained energy release. The key to achieving this is to ensure that you eat a wide variety of proteins that include vegetable sources as well as the more traditional meat, fish and dairy sources.

Maximise Your Protein Intake	
Increase Protein Frequency	Eat protein with each meal and snack, including breakfast. During times of stress, increase your protein intake.
Eat Good Quality Animal Protein	Include lean meat, fish, fowl, eggs and dairy, as these are high quality proteins.
Include Vegetable Protein	Beans, soya, legumes peas, nuts and seeds. Small amounts are also found in seeds, grains, vegetables and fruits.
Snacks to Include Protein	These can be simple as spreading humous or peanut butter on a cracker or eating nuts with fruit.

Sugar Overload

The Western world is in a 'sugar crises'. Sugar is consumed in alarming quantities every day leading to energy and mood fluctuations, weight problems, hormonal imbalances and other health conditions. It is everywhere and often you don't even realise that you are consuming it. Large amounts of added sugar can be hidden in foods such as bread, canned soups and vegetables, pasta sauce, margarine, frozen dinners, fast food, soy sauce, and ketchup.

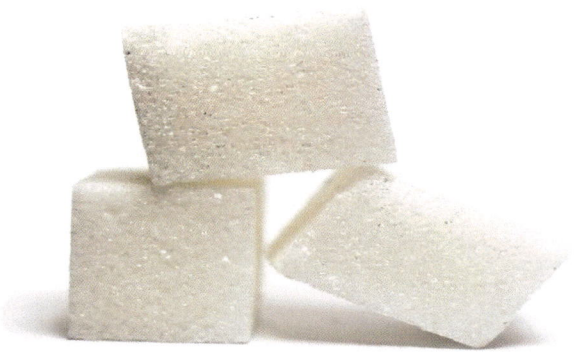

Source: www.pixabay.com

Be especially careful of added fructose. Since the 1970s, there has been a steady increase in the amount of fructose used in processed foods, either as high-fructose corn syrup or sucrose (a mixture of glucose and fructose). It is normally used as a sweetener in soft drinks, breakfast cereals, baked goods, condiments and prepared desserts. Not only does this added fructose provide a large number of calories; compared to glucose, fructose is preferentially metabolised to fat rather than burnt as a fuel for energy.[240]

Such are the health concerns about added fructose, that it has also now been implicated in the epidemics of obesity, type-2 diabetes, insulin resistance, hypertension, central body fat and the metabolic syndrome.[241] However, fructose found naturally in fruit will be accompanied by fibre and other nutrients that will slow down the digestion and reduce blood sugar spikes. **The key to controlling sugar is to prepare your own food and to plan your diet around fibre-rich vegetables, fruits, whole grains, lean proteins and good fats.** Move away from the processed and ready-made foods, limit your sweet treats and learn to read the 'hidden' sugar on food labels.

Limit Your Sugar	
Avoid Sugary Drinks	Such as coke and other soft drinks as these can contain up to 10 teaspoons of sugar. Try sparkling water with lemon or a splash of fruit juice.
Go for Natural Sweetness	Use naturally sweet food such as fruit, organic honey, agave nectar, or natural nut butters to satisfy your sweet tooth.
Read Food Labels	Sugar is often disguised using terms such as maple syrup, corn syrup/sweetener, honey, molasses, brown rice syrup, fruit juice concentrates, maltodextrin/dextrin, dextrose, fructose, glucose, maltose or sucrose. Learn to read the labels and avoid the hidden sugars.

Food Timing

Food timing is an important signal for setting the rhythm of the metabolic clock.[242] Anticipatory behaviour, even when food is restricted, occurs just before scheduled meal times.[243] This is characterised by changes to body temperature, hormones and enzymes; which prepare the body for the anticipated food intake.[244] The metabolic clock is linked to the central clock that stays locked to the light-dark cycle but when eating occurs outside of the normal eating times, the metabolic clock becomes dysregulated from the central clock.[245] Hence, ghrelin (the hunger hormone) will be secreted in anticipation of feeding, regardless of whether it is night or day.[246] If you find yourself eating all of the time or at irregular hours, then try to establish a regular daily eating pattern to re-set your metabolic clock. And if you are skipping meals, your metabolic clock wil still be ticking, so make sure that you eat your main meals of breakfast, lunch and dinner.

Key Action Points

Tip 1	• Set yourself up for success.
Tip 2	• Moderation and balance.
Tip 3	• Reconnect with food.
Tip 4	• Eat rainbow fruit and vegetables.
Tip 5	• Eat complex carbs and whole grains.
Tip 6	• Eat good fats and avoid the bad.
Tip 7	• Eat protein with every meal.
Tip 8	• Limit your sugar intake.

Chapter 11: The Case for Supplements

Hype or Help?

We are repeatedly told that you will get all the nutrients that you need from a healthy diet and that you do not require nutritional supplements. But is this true? Certainly, supplements should be as the name suggests - 'supplemental' to diet - and that diet should always be the starting point. However, many people are confused about what a proper healthy diet is for them, whilst multiple other factors can lead to an increased need for additional nutrients over and above that which can be supplied by food alone. Everyone is individual and lifestyle factors vary from individual to individual. However, nutritional supplements can help to support a healthy lifestyle for many people.

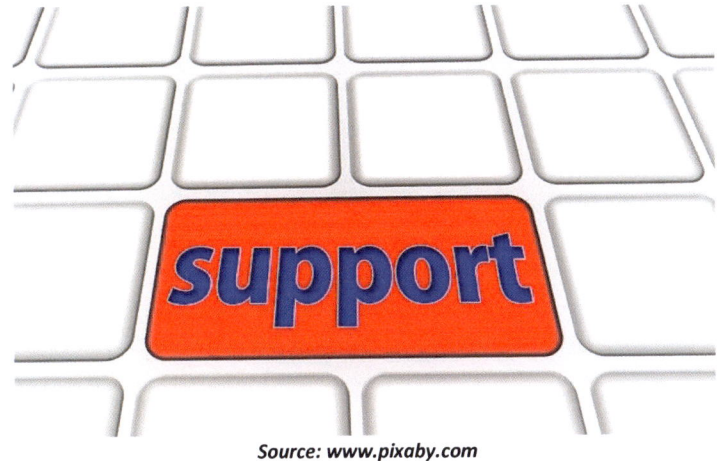

Source: www.pixaby.com

The Food Chain Supply

Farming practices have changed over the centuries. Gone are the days when fields were routinely left fallow to restore soil fertility. Now, with intensive farming, plants are repeatedly grown on the same land, which causes the soil to lose nutrients faster than they can be replaced. Fertiliser helps nourish plants so that they survive but will not replace the lost nutrients from the soil. It has been estimated that such practices results in up to **75% fewer micronutrients**.[247] Furthermore, once harvested those plants then sit on trucks, shelves, shop counters and in your fridge for weeks before being eaten – leading to a further deterioration in the nutrient content.

Other practices also contribute to reduced nutrient content. Animals that are grain-fed, rather than grass-fed, acquire a lower nutrient content from the grain than they would otherwise from the grass. Meat from such animals tends to be very low in vitamins, minerals, fatty acids and antioxidants. Then there is the food processing element. Food is refined and processed so that it lasts longer but, in so doing, vital nutrients are either stripped from the food or destroyed, thereby depleting the foodstuff even further. Hence, the food that we eat now is far inferior in micronutrient content to the food eaten by our ancestors.

Environmental Toxin Exposure

Environmental toxins are on the increase and they are impossible to avoid. You will be taking in these toxins on a daily basis from the food that you eat, the water that you drink, the air that you breathe and the environment around you. These toxins are harmful to your body so the body will try to eliminate them through its natural detoxification pathways. However, those pathways require nutrients to function, so the more toxins that you take in the more nutrients that you will require to upregulate their detoxification. Below is a list of some of the most common environmental toxins and their major sources:[248]

Environmental Toxin	Major Sources
PCBs (polychlorinated diphenyls)	Plastics, farm-raised salmon
Pesticides	Fruits, vegetables, commercial meats
Mould & fungal toxins	Contaminated buildings, peanuts, alcohol
Phthalates	Plastic wraps, bottles, food storage containers
VOCs (volatile organic compounds)	Drinking water, carpets, paints, deodorants, cleaning fluids, air fresheners
Dioxins	Commercial animal fats
Heavy metals (arsenic, mercury, lead, aluminium, cadmium)	Drinking water, fish, vaccines, pesticides, deodorants, dental amalgams, smoking
Chlorine	Drinking water, household cleaners
Xenoestrogens	Plastics, water supply, petroleum products

Age, Exercise and Stress

There is no doubt that physiological changes also impact nutrient requirements. Nutrient absorption often declines with age (for a variety of reasons), whilst both exercise and stress upregulate the same pathways that facilitates the immediate availability of greater energy resources. Like all biochemical pathways in the body, micronutrients are required for proper function of the energy generating pathways. The more frequent the exercise and stress, the more nutrients that will be needed to provide the energy required to meet the demands.

Misleading News Stories

Scaremongering in the press about the use of supplements appears to be on the increase and leads to confusion for consumers as to safety and viability. Often study results are misinterpreted or misreported in the press and, without access to the original research paper or understanding the context of the claim, it is hard for the average person to know the truth. Conversely, numerous reports on how insufficient nutrient intake contributes towards many health problems, as well as the impressive health benefits that result from regular dietary micronutrient supplementation, are less publicised and often completely ignored.

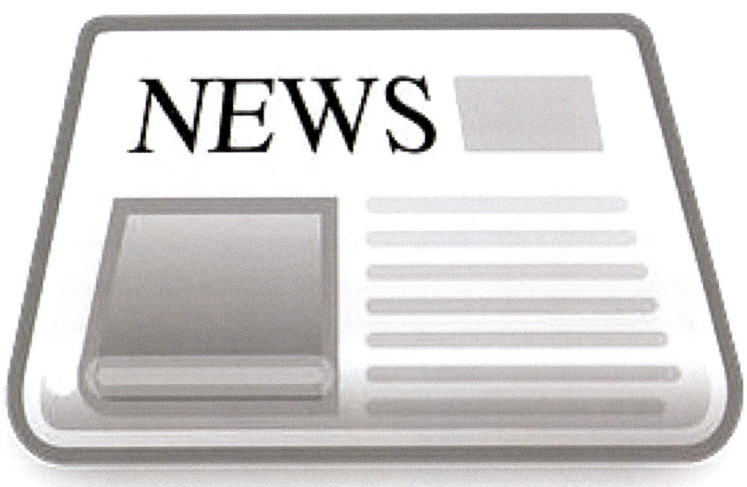

Source: www.pixabay.com

Which? Magazine (a UK health consumer magazine) provides a case in point. In September 2013, it published an article titled *"Don't believe the hype – people are wasting money on unnecessary food supplements"*, which was widely covered by the UK media. In this article, they suggested that only a minority of people required nutritional supplements and that people may be wasting money unnecessarily as a result of manufacturers making misleading claims on their products. The background context to this was the introduction into UK law in December 2012 of the European Union (EU) Health Claims Regulations, whereby UK manufacturers were required to only make health claims with regards to nutrients that were approved by the European Food Safety Authority (EFSA).

In response to this article, the **UK Health Food Manufacturers' Association (HFMA)** issued a press release rebutting these claims (not widely reported by the media), which included the following comments:

"This report is inaccurate as it infers that manufacturers are misleading their customers, which is simply not true. Just because a certain ingredient does not have an EFSA-approved claim, does not mean that it does not have a beneficial effect. The huge quantity of claims that have been 'rejected' is largely a result of EFSA applying an inappropriate pharmaceutical-style assessment to generic health maintenance claims on food ingredients; an approach usually used for assessing illness-related claims on drugs, which are completely different. Consequently, the list of unauthorised claims ignores the genuine value and evidence behind these products. The report also ignores the significant efforts by UK manufacturers' to comply with the regulation as well as still provide factual information about what their products do and how they work.

The Scientific Evidence

Overwhelming basic science and experimental data support the use of nutritional supplements for the prevention of disease and the support of optimal health. Extensive literature reviews in respected peer-reviewed medical journals[249][250] also support this view. Gold standard randomised controlled interventionist trials that prove cause and effect have provided positive outcomes in multiple health conditions. However, there are some studies that have shown harm rather than benefit. Mainly, those studies were flawed because the studies themselves were designed like drugs studies, whereby a high dose of a particular nutrient is used to see what happens without taking into account that nutrients work together in synergy and not alone. Nutrients are not drugs and will not function like drugs.

Over and above the individual studies, it is universally recognised that taking any of the micronutrients (vitamins and minerals) in high doses can be toxic. As the 'micronutrient' name suggests, these nutrients are required in small quantities by the body. Consequently, various authoritative bodies *(HFMA, Institute of Medicine, US Food & Nutrition Board, EU Scientific Committee for Food)* recommend an **Upper Safe Level (USL)** for the dosage of individual nutrients based on available scientific studies that have shown those levels to be safe. It is within these safe recommendations that supplement manufacturers and those giving supplement advice operate. For the avoidance of doubt, these USLs are usually way above the country **RDAs *(recommended daily allowances)*;** which are, in effect, the *minimal dosage* required to prevent the occurrence of recognised nutritional-related diseases (such as scurvy), rather than the recommend amount for optimal health.

Statistics

To put all of this into context, let's take a look at some statistics: The HFMA has stated that figures published by the *UK Food Standard Agency* showed that there were only 11 cases of adverse reactions to supplements in the past 11 years, most of them in the category of low risk to health. Likewise, in the US, not one person died as a result of taking vitamins in 2010.[251] In contrast, deaths from prescription drug overdoses have been rising steadily over the past 20 years, resulting in it now being the leading cause of death in the US.[252] In 2013, there were **22,767 deaths in the US attributed to unintentional pharmaceutical drug overdose** (especially opioid pain relievers or prescription painkillers).[253]

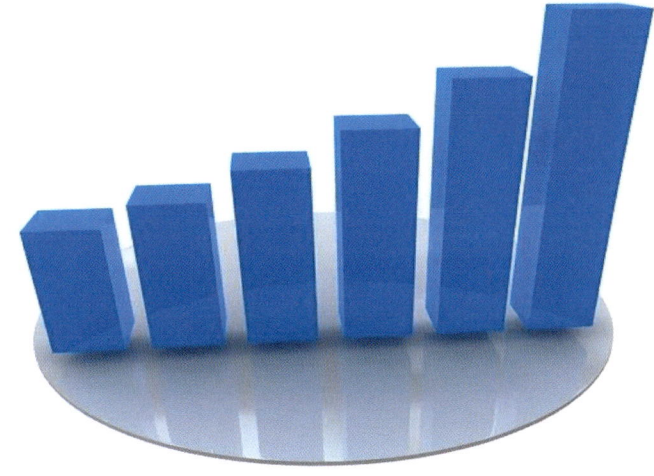

Source: www.pixabay.com

In comparison, nutritional supplementation is very safe. However, it is important to note that **nutrient-drug interactions** are well documented and need to be considered on an individual basis. According to **Dr Aleksandra Neidzwieki** (a well renowned biochemist who has worked directly with two Nobel Laureates and is the author of 60 original research papers):[254]

> *"Ultimately, the reality that the mass media is not sharing with you is that vitamins are dangerous ONLY to the pharmaceutical business, which sees that they undermine its disease market and reduces the outlet for dangerous patented pharmaceutical drug compounds".*

The Supplement Market

Millions of us take dietary supplements hoping to achieve good health, ease our illnesses or defy ageing. Recent years have seen a massive boom in supplement use as products that were once the preserves of specialist health food stores have become available alongside our groceries in the supermarket and on the internet. As availability has grown, so have sales. In 2009, the UK market for dietary supplements and vitamins was worth more than £670 million.[255] In the US, projected sales figures for 2018 are $16.4 billion.[256] Today, the production of dietary supplements is big business, which has spawned a huge range of dietary supplements that makes the area something of a minefield for consumers.

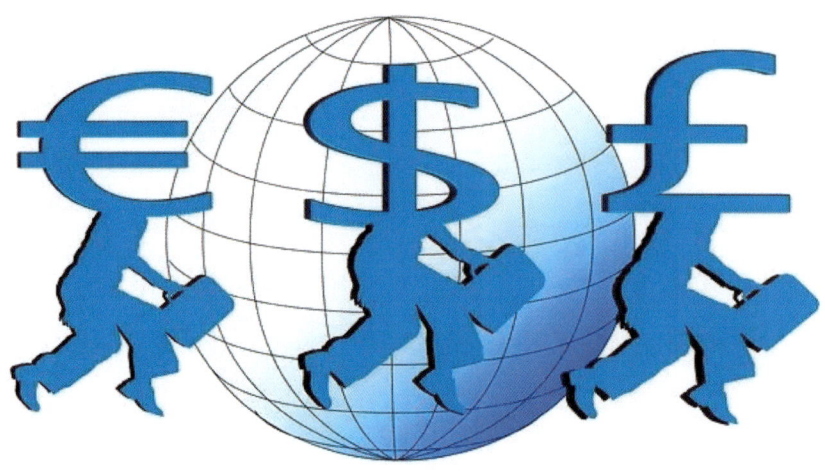

Source: www.pixabay.com

Natural vs Synthetic Supplements

The vast majority of the supplements that you encounter are likely to be synthetic. Many natural nutrients are unable to meet the requirements of modern manufacturing in terms of volume, consistency and quality; whilst nutrients in the natural forms tend to be sensitive to outside influences, such as heat and light, and can easily be destroyed by the very act of extraction. Manufacturers who synthesise vitamins are able to modify their forms so that they are more stable and can be used for a variety of applications. Pure, synthetic vitamins are far more concentrated than many natural forms of nutrients, which makes them important for the manufacture of capsules and tablets. Legally, products also have to have a guaranteed potency, purity and shelf life, which make synthetic nutrients easier to control.

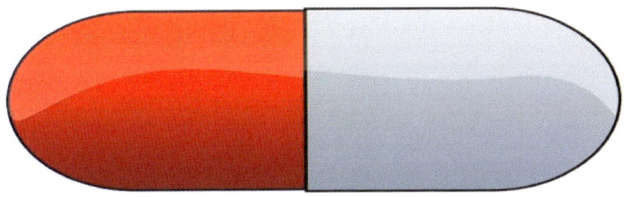

Source: www.pixabay.com

Despite the above, a *'natural alternatives'* market continues to thrive, with more and more sophisticated formulas coming onto the market. These include *'food state'* nutrients, where the vitamin or mineral is added to a food during manufacture to complex with the food. The orthodox view is that synthesised vitamins are identical to those found in food. Chemically, that is true, but the synthetic molecules have a slightly different twist that makes them structurally different. This rotational difference becomes apparent if a polarized light is passed through the molecule. For a natural vitamin, the light will always bend to the **right** so the letter **"d"** *("dextro", which means right)* will appear on the label; whereas for synthetic vitamins, the light will split into two parts (one part right, the other left), so the letters **"dl"** *("dextro" (right) and "levo" (left))* will be ascribed to it.

Although these structural differences exist, there appears to be no substantial evidence to show that the bioavailability of the synthetic and natural forms is different, with the exception of vitamin E. Studies have shown that synthetic vitamin E (dl-alpha tocopherol) is not retained by the body as readily as the natural vitamin (d-alpha tocopherol).[257] Hence, it is less bioavailable. Good supplement manufacturers will take into account absorption factors and will often include co-factors that aid absorption in nature, such as vitamin C with bioflavonoids. As the vast majority of the scientific nutrition intervention studies will have used synthetic versions of the nutrients which have been shown to be safe, the overwhelming health benefits found from such use is a very strong argument in their favour.

Supplement Brands

There are a vast amount of supplement brands on the market, making your choice of product difficult. Be aware that the cheaper the product, the more likely it is that inferior ingredients will have been used; that there will be a greater amount of excipients; and that the greater the likelihood of poor absorption. **You are not just what you eat but also what you absorb.** Check with a reputable health food retailer or a qualified nutritionist for the best local brands.

Chapter 12: Specific Supplements

Health Foundation Supplements

The Basics

There are four basic supplements that can be thought of as the foundations for health, irrespective of the health condition, but which are also fundamentally important to energy-related conditions. They are as follows:

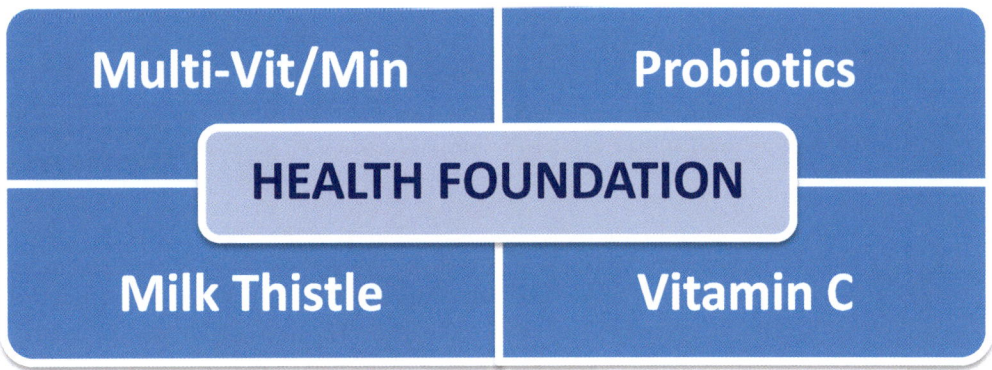

Multi-Vitamins and Minerals

Additional regular micro-nutrient support would seem prudent in light of the reduced nutrient content in modern foods and the increased need for their utilisation in a wide range of scenarios. A 2014 review paper has revealed that the typical American diet bears little resemblance to what experts recommend in terms of micro-nutrient content; and, that with time, such deficiencies may lead to serious health issues.[258] Conversely, such nutritional inadequacies are far less common among users of multi-vitamins and minerals.[259] It is now recognised that the use of such supplements can be instrumental in filling nutritional gaps,[260] including in populations where the food supply is relatively bountiful and balanced.[261]

The energy generating process, like other biochemical systems, requires micro-nutrient sufficiency for energy to be generated effectively. This is because specific micro-nutrients act as co-factors for the mitochondrial enzymes that produce energy. However, some of those key co-factors can often be lacking in today's modern diet.

KEY Mitochondrial Co-Factors	
Magnesium	B-Vitamins
Iron	Manganese
Sulphur	Copper
CoQ10	Selenium

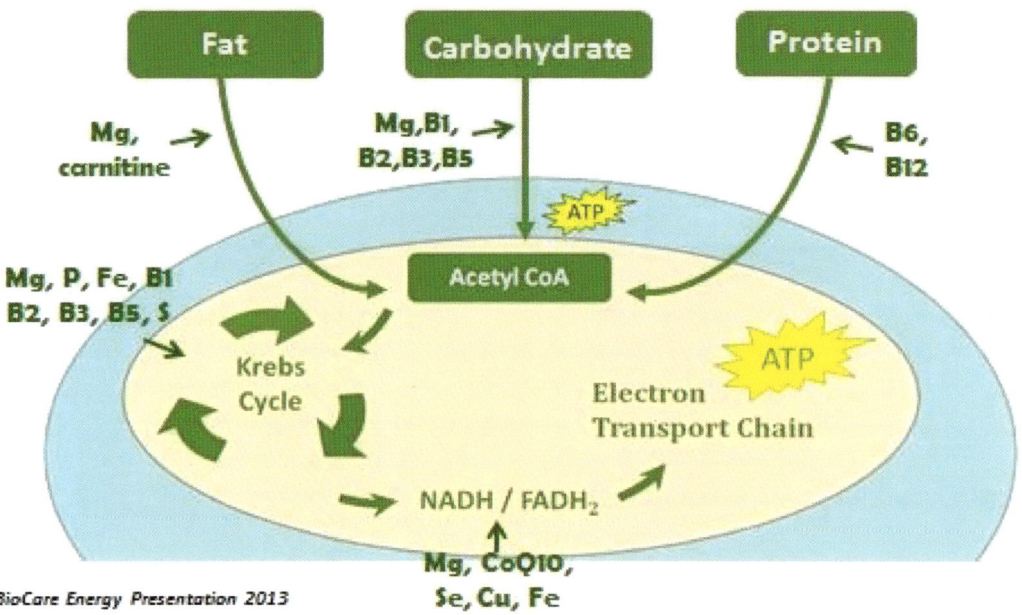

Look for a multi that has broad coverage of the main vitamins and minerals. Bioavailability is paramount for maximum absorption – minerals, in particular, tend to be poorly absorbed – so be aware of the different nutrient binding substances, called **chelates,** which can affect absorption. Organic acid chelates (such as *citric acid/citrate, malic acid/malate or picolinic acid/picolinate*) are much better absorbed than non-organic forms (such as *carbonates, oxides or sulphates*), which can sometimes promote side-effects such as gastrointestinal distress. Plus, the fat-soluble nutrients (*vitamins A, D, E and K)* are better absorbed if they are emulsified. Try and avoid common allergens (such as gluten or dairy derivatives), as well as high levels of excipients (additives such as colourings and fillers). Dosage-wise, choose an optimum level product as it will likely be above the country *RDA (and* within the *Upper Safe Levels).* Seek advice from a health practitioner, health store or the manufacturer if you are unsure of the dosage.

Multi dosage • Optimum level/day

Probiotics

A key connection exists between gut micro-flora, energy production and metabolic-related disorders.[262] The gut microbiota has now been found to exert a significant role in the pathogenesis of **metabolic syndrom** and the related **non-alcoholic fatty liver disease (NAFLD)**.[263] The complex balance of 'good' and 'bad' bacteria in the gut can affect metabolic balance by modulating energy absorption, gut motility, appetite, glucose and lipid metabolism, as well as liver fat storage.[264] Gut microflora imbalance can impair the gut barrier, leading to translocation of bacterial fragments from the gut into the liver (via the portal blood system).[265] This can result in **metabolic endotoxemia** - toxicity caused by the release of toxic substances from bacterial cell walls upon rupture or disintegration - and systemic inflammation from the interaction of the bacteria with the immune system.[266]

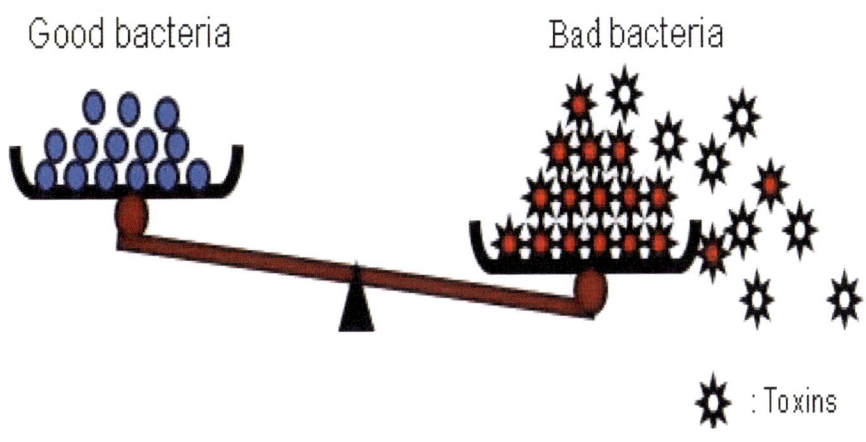

Source: www.biogif.com

The main friendly ("good") bacteria in the gut are lactobacillus and bifidobacteria. The presence of these two types of bacteria has been found to decrease endotoxemia and inflammation, reduce intestinal permeability and improve glucose tolerance.[267] They exert their effects by enhancing the integrity of the gut barrier and preventing bacterial translocation.[268] Several studies on metabolic syndrome have demonstrated that *probiotics (live good bacteria)* containing lactobacillus and bifidobacterium strains can promote weight loss, reduce central fat, improve glucose tolerance and modulate inflammation.[269] Encouraging results are now also emerging for the use of probiotics in NAFLD.[270]

Good bacteria
- Lactobacillus acidophilus
- Bifidobacteria bifidum

The use of probiotics for supporting gut health is now common place. The direct effects of probiotics in the GI tract are well documented, whilst there is a now a large amount of promising data on the preventive and therapeutic effects of probiotics in several diseases,[271] including metabolic disorders.[272] The sheer weight of evidence in their favour is currently impacting the medical establishment with many doctors now advocating their use for GI disorders. Few clinical studies demonstrate a significant benefit where a dose of less than **10 billion** bacteria has been used. Look for a brand that typically offers 10 billion or more per capsule containing both lactobacillus and bifdobacteria and that require refrigeration. Unrefrigerated probiotics will have compromised potency because of natural heat-related decomposition.

Probiotics dosage • 10 billion/day

Milk Thistle (AKA Silymarin)

Silymarin (a standardized extract of milk thistle) has a long tradition over the centuries as a liver-protective herbal remedy, and for over 30 years it has been used clinically in Europe and Asia for the treatment of liver diseases.[273] The liver plays a central role in metabolic energy homeostasis, detoxification and immunity[274] - as well as a wide range of other functions - and can be likened to a power and sewage/filtration plant.[275] Its main functions are to take up nutrients, store them and provide them to other organs; in addition to clearing potentially damaging substances from the circulation. Due to its roles, it is frequently exposed to various insults which can cause cell death and hepatic dysfunction, although it has a remarkable ability to self-repair and regenerate after injury.[276] It is the only internal organ capable of natural regeneration of lost tissue – as little as 25% of a liver can regenerate into a whole liver.[277]

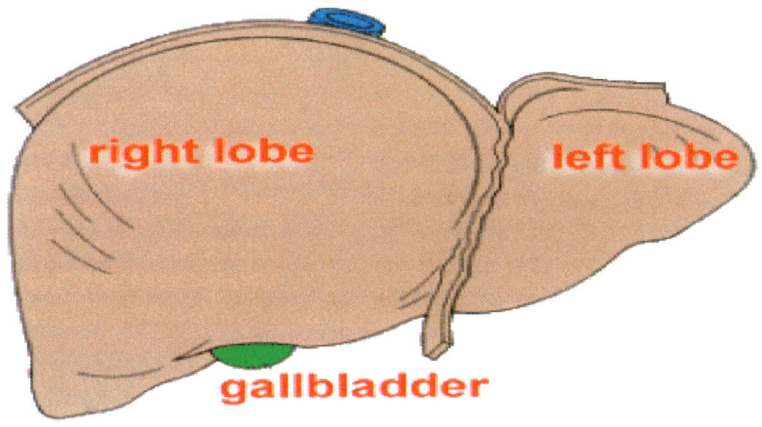

Source: www.le.ac.uk

The process of aging predisposes the liver to functional and structural impairment and metabolic risk, via decreased antioxidant levels and increased levels of inflammatory markers and free radicals.[278] Ultimately, this can lead to liver disease. The most common liver disease in the world, affecting one-third of the population, is ***non-alcoholic fatty liver disease (NAFLD),*** which is the leading cause of liver injury.[279] It is a modern day medical condition associated with aging[280] and pathological energy-disorder related conditions, including obesity, type-2 diabetes and the metabolic syndrome.[281] NAFLD is characterised by fat accumulation in the liver,[282] inflammation, insulin resistance, oxidative stress (an imbalance of free radicals and antioxidants) and fibrosis.[283]

The protective effects of milk thistle results from its anti-inflammatory and anti-fibrotic properties, together with its ability to modulate the immune response, protect cell membranes, and promote liver tissue regeneration.[284] With the rise of metabolic related disorders and an aging population, research has once again focused on the liver protective effects of milk thistle. Recent study reviews have now shown the effectiveness of milk thistle extract in targeting the pathological effects of NAFLD,[285] [286] whilst clinical trials have confirmed that silymarin is currently the best medication for NAFLD.[287] Evidence shows that a **dosage of 140 mg/day of silymarin** is effective in the treatment of NAFLD.[288] However, be aware that there is very little commercial standardisation as to levels of silymarin extract. Most commercial products range from 20-40% extraction level. Aim for the highest extraction level that you can find. The percentage extraction will be found on the label of the supplement.

Silymarin dosage	• 140 mg/day

Vitamin C (AKA Ascorbic Acid)

Vitamin C is probably best known for its antioxidant properties that enable it to protect cells and tissues from damage due to *free radicals* (unstable molecules) generated by inflammation and metabolic by-products.[289] But it is also involved in the regulation of both circulating and liver lipid homeostasis.[290] An association has now been found between poor vitamin C status and the propagation of lifestyle associated diseases.[291] About 10-20% of the Western population can be diagnosed with vitamin C deficiency - although this may be higher in certain sub-groups - and that poor vitamin C status is associated with increased all-cause mortality.[292] An inverse correlation also exists between vitamin C status, BMI (body mass index) and body fat percentage;[293] with an apparent link between obesity, metabolic syndrome and NAFLD.[294]

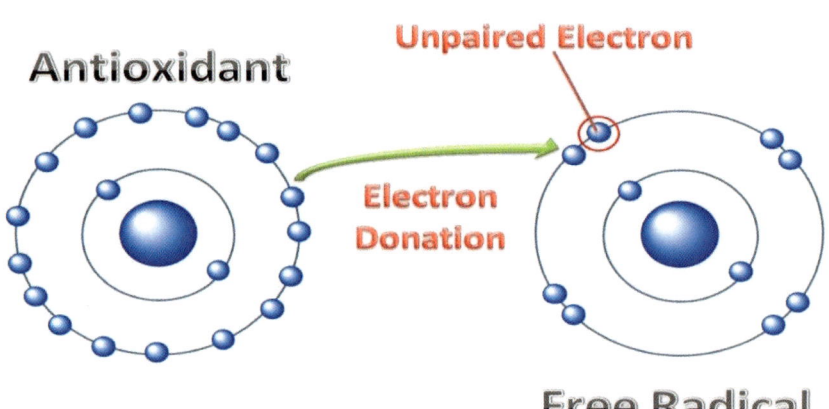

Source: www.healthyprotocols.net

Given that uncontrolled inflammation is a key pathogenic mechanism in many diseases,[295] it is not surprising that numerous studies have demonstrated that vitamin C supplementation decreases the risk of a wide range of pathologies.[296] This includes *atherosclerosis* (hardening of the arteries) - a disease initially of inflammation and then subsequent oxidative damage[297] –

that is linked with the metabolic syndrome.[298] Atherosclerosis is the single biggest cause of death in the developed world, accounting for 1 in 3 of all deaths.[299] Worldwide, it accounts for 17.3 million deaths per year and is expected to grow to more than 23.6 million by 2030.[300]

Many important enzyme reactions also require vitamin C as a co-factor, including the synthesis of nor-adrenaline (stress hormone), carnitine (fat transporter), cholesterol (steroid hormone precursor), amino acids, and collagen (main structural protein of connective tissue).[301] Because collagen is so important to the connective tissue network, vitamin C deficiency results in a weakening of the tissue leading to bleeding and blood loss[302] - a condition called scurvy, which is more synonymous with the seafarers of the 17th century. However, such is its deficiency today resulting from a 'junk food' diet that the UK has recently reported a sharp rise in childhood scurvy cases.

To ensure an optimal intake of vitamin C, the current literature indicates supplementation of **1,000 mg/day**, accompanied by a diet rich in fruits and vegetables.[303] This level has also been shown to reduce the concentration of circulating fats and other metabolic parameters, including blood sugar levels.[304] Look for a vitamin C supplement that is buffered with magnesium or potassium to reduce the acidity and improve stomach tolerance.

Vitamin C dosage	• 1,000 mg/day

Energy Specific Supplements

Cellular Energy Nutrients

In addition to or instead of the general foundation supplements, more specific supplements can be used to target the energy-generating process of the body to raise the energy levels at times of need. Bear in mind that you will still need to have a proper health foundation, which can be achieved by following the advice on nutrition and lifestyle. However, there are times when you need to just raise your energy levels before tackling the basics and there are times when you need specific energy support to cope with increased metabolic demand. The following nutrients are significant for their roles in energy generation:

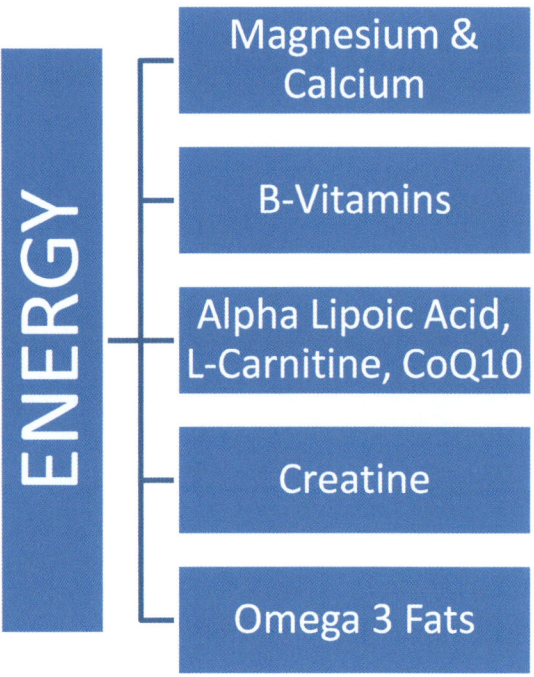

Many supplement manufacturers now combine these ingredients into one or more complex formulas, so there will generally be no need to purchase these individually.

Magnesium and Calcium

Magnesium (Mg) and calcium (Ca) work together as a pair and, therefore, you should always consider both nutrients when supplementing. **Magnesium plays a central role in energy metabolism and the production of ATP energy.**[305] It is essential to the ATP molecule itself as ATP must be bound to a magnesium ion to be biologically active; so technically, ATP should be called **Mg-ATP**.[306] It is also a co-factor for over 300 metabolic reactions in the body,[307] helps to stabilise mitochondrial membranes,[308] and plays a critical role in maintaining normal nerve and muscle function, as well as glucose and insulin metabolism.[309] Low levels are associated with increased inflammation, a risk of type 2 diabetes, cardiovascular disease,[310] and metabolic syndrome;[311] as well as a number of other chronic diseases.[312]

Magnesium supplementation can prevent blood sugar levels from falling excessively,[313] reduce HPA over-activity, improve sleep patterns[314] and insulin resistance,[315] and at dosages of **200-**

450 mg/day can reduce symptoms of metabolic syndrome. In athletes, dosages of 350 mg/day have been found to improve anaerobic alactic metabolism[316] - the phosphocreatine system that rapidly regenerates ATP to produce massive bursts of energy in very short periods of time where there is a high metabolic demand.

Mg dosage	• 200-450 mg/day

Calcium, although known to be central to nerve and muscle function,[317] has also recently been identified as being integral to cellular energy production through regulation of enzymes involved in ATP synthesis.[318] It provides a fundamental control system regulating ATP production through an ongoing shuttling of calcium to the mitochondria from the endoplasmic reticulum (a cellular organelle).[319] However, under stress conditions, it is magnesium that controls the activation of the calcium-dependent enzymes, and hence calcium's signalling and metabolic functions.[320]

Low calcium levels are linked to an increased prevalence of total and/or abdominal obesity, insulin resistance, type 2 diabetes and high blood pressure.[321] Of great importance is the ratio between calcium and magnesium intake because they antagonize each other in intestinal absorption.[322] A ***calcium-magnesium ratio of 1.7 : 2.5*** has been shown to reduce inflammation and cardiovascular risks; whilst in the elderly with type-2 diabetes, this ratio has been shown to be 2.0 : 2.5.[323] If you take a magnesium supplement, then also take a calcium supplement. It is probably easiest to ***use an approximate ratio of Ca : Mg of 2.0 : 2.5.***

Ca dosage	• 160-360 mg/day

B Vitamins

The B vitamins, in particular, serve an important role as cofactors in energy metabolism and as such are essential for maintaining mitochondrial function.[324] They can also improve stress[325] and reduce anxiety and strain.[326] Energy metabolism consists of a series of enzymatic reactions that convert macronutrients into ATP. However, they do not work in isolation – they require several vitamins to help them carry out the metabolic reactions. Each of the B vitamins (thiamine (B1), riboflavin (B2), niacin (B3), pantothenic acid (B5), pyridoxal (B6), biotin (B7), cobalamine (B12) and folic acid) serves as a cofactor in various aspects of carbohydrate, fat and protein metabolism.[327] Deficiency of any one of them can restrict the rate of reaction and compromise mitochondrial function.[328] Because the B-group vitamins work together, it is always best to supplement them together in a complex form. Look for a **B-50s formula** containing a minimum of 400 mcg folic acid, 50 mcg B12 and biotin, and 50 mg of all the other B vitamins.

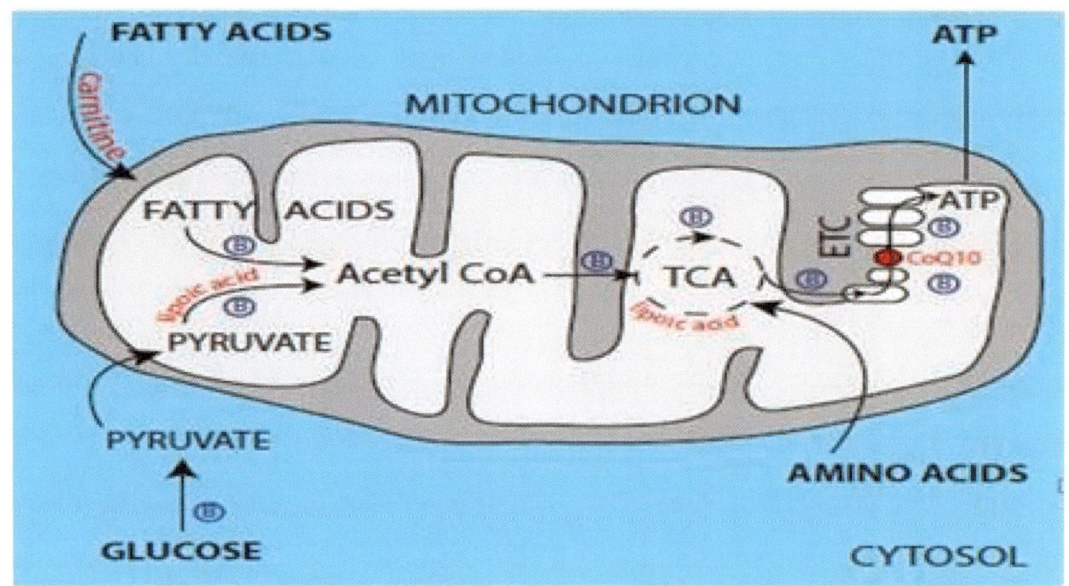

B vitamins (B) operate at sites all along the entire path of macronutrient breakdown (black arrows). Sites of lipoic acid, CoQ10 and carnitine involvement are highlighted in red. TCA= tricarboxylic acid cycle (AKA Kreb's/citric acid cycle); ETC=electron transport chain.
Angelo G (2013). http://pi.oregonstate.edu/ss13/metabolims.html

B-vitamins dosage
- Most = 50 mg/day
- Folic acid = 400 mcg/day
- B12/biotin = 50 mcg/day

Alpha-Lipoic Acid, L-Carnitine and CoQ10

In addition to the B vitamins, other nutrients also operate in energy metabolism. In particular, *alpha-lipoic acid* (derived from a short-chain fatty acid); *L-carnitine* (derived from the amino acids lysine and methionine); and *CoQ10* (a vitamin-like fat soluble molecule). Each participates in different aspects of cellular energy production:

Alpha-lipoic acid (ALA) (*AKA lipoic acid*) is a co-factor in enzymes involved in glucose breakdown and the Krebs cycle in the mitochondria;[329] as well as a powerful antioxidant involved in quenching free radicals and regenerating glutathione (main intra-cellular antioxidant) and vitamins C and E.[330] However, it also has other functions that make it special to supporting energy production. In particular, it activates the expression of the cellular energy enzyme **AMPK (adenosine monophosphate-activated protein kinase)**[331] and modulates gene expression in key regulatory enzymes in glucose and lipid metabolism[332] via inducing **PPARs (*peroxisome proliferator-activated receptors*)**.[333]

AMPK functions as a fuel sensor in the cell and is activated when cellular energy is depleted.[334] It also plays a critical role in modulating gene expression via inducing PPARs,[335] which are direct regulators of core-clock genes that regulate metabolism and energy homeostasis.[336] AMPK activation inhibits the energy-consuming biosynthetic pathways that store energy and activates the catabolic pathways that produce ATP by increasing glucose uptake and fat breakdown.[337] PPARs are now believed to be the molecular links between the circadian rhythm and energy metabolism.[338]

As a therapeutic agent, the beneficial effects of ALA have now been demonstrated in a number of experimental and clinical studies for a diverse spectrum of diseases from metabolic disorders, such as metabolic syndrome, to heavy metal poisoning.[339] In particular, it can improve insulin sensitivity and reduce fat accumulation.[340] Increases in energy expenditure and reduced plasma glucose, insulin, free fatty acids and leptin have all been demonstrated in rats;[341] whilst in humans, reduced body weight has been found in obese diabetics at a dosage of 1,800 mg/day.[342] For general therapeutic purposes, **600 mg/day** appears to be the maximum effective dose.[343]

ALA dosage	• 600 mg/day

L-carnitine

Carnitine plays a vital role in energy production and fatty acid metabolism[344] by transporting fats into the mitochondria for breakdown.[345] It also exports excess lipids[346] and xenobiotics (foreign substances)[347] from the mitochondria to protect mitochondrial function. Without carnitine, the inner mitochondrial membrane would be impermeable to fats,[348] thereby preventing dietary lipids being used as an energy source and leading to an accumulation of lipids and obesity.[349] Sustained metabolic stress increases its requirements,[350] whilst carnitine decline is a common trait of insulin resistant states such as diet-induced obesity.[351] Deficiency generally occurs due to, or in association with, other disorders such as defects in fatty acid metabolism.[352]

Evidence now suggests that a carnitine controlled enzyme in the brain hypothalamus - **CPT-1c (carnitine palmitoyl transferase-1c)** – plays an important regulatory role in energy homeostasis.[353] The **arcuate nucleus (ARC)** of the hypothalamus has emerged as an integral regulator of whole-body energy homeostasis that integrates hormonal, energy substrate and neuronal cues.[354] Control is exerted via the central nervous system (CNS) through the regulation of feeding behaviour and satiety[355] via the activation or inhibition of AMPK[356] - the fuel-sensing enzyme that detects energy status[357] and modulates feeding and energy homeostasis.[358] Hypothalamic fatty acid metabolism plays a key role[359] - it is the glucose flux into fatty acid synthesis that mediates the satiety response[360] - whilst CPT-1c acts as the nutrient sensing signalling mechanism[361] that integrates carbohydrate and lipid nutrient sensing to regulate feeding behaviour.[362]

Carnitine supplementation has been shown to enhance glucose utilisation, lower insulin resistance[363] and has been associated with a significant reduction in all-cause mortality and some cardiovascular conditions.[364] The favourable effects in cardiovascular conditions may stem from fats being the primary energy source of the heart.[365] However, the bioavailability of carnitine from oral supplements is very low, ranging from 5-18%[366] - mainly because a significant proportion is metabolised by gut microbiota prior to absorption.[367] Hence, high doses are generally required. Supplementation at **3 g/day** has been shown to be the optimal level for reducing all-cause mortality risk.[368] **Acetyl-L-carnitine** is the most bioavailable form.[369]

Acetyl-L-carnitine dosage	• 3 g/day

CoQ10 (Co-enzyme Q10)

CoQ10 or **ubiquinone** is a fat soluble molecule present in all tissues and cells and is located in all cell membranes, mainly in the inner mitochondrial membrane.[370] It plays a critical role in energy production as an integral component of the *Electron Transport Chain* – the final part of mitochondrial energy production – where it is reduced to **ubiquinol** and acts as an electron shuttle during the formation of ATP.[371] It is also a potent regulator of multiple genes (including cell signalling, metabolism and nutrient transport);[372] and induces PPAR expression via a calcium-mediated AMPK signalling pathway - which suppresses lipogenesis and adipogenesis, whilst increasing fatty acid oxidation.[373] In its **ubiquinol** form, it also functions as a lipid-soluble antioxidant in cell membranes,[374] where it acts with vitamin E to prevent membrane damage.[375]

Alterations of mitochondrial enzymes involved in CoQ10 mechanisms have been found to occur in metabolic conditions, cardiovascular disease, oxidative stress and aging.[376] High energy production increases the requirements of mitochondrial CoQ10,[377] whilst deficiency may disrupt several vital cellular functions.[378] Increased mitochondrial CoQ10 content results in improved oxygen consumption and ATP production.[379] Supplementation has been found to reduce blood glucose and blood pressure, and may improve certain cardiovascular conditions.[380] However, supplementation appears more effective alongside alpha-lipoic acid, where a synergistic action occurs; leading to increased inducement of PPARs, improved stress response and significantly increased cellular glutathione levels.[381] This synergistic effect may be linked to the ability of alpha-lipoic acid to reduce ubiquinone to ubiquinol.[382]

Therapeutic dosages of CoQ10 range from **100-300 mg/day**. However, absorption is generally poor due to its lack of solubility in water.[383] For better bioavailability, look for a supplement in ubiquinone form that is dissolved in oil and emulsified, and take alongside a fatty meal as bile is needed for absorption. Doses higher than 100 mg/day should be split into divided doses as absorption decreases with increasing supplemental dose.[384]

CoQ10 dosage	100-300 mg/day

Creatine

Creatine is a naturally occurring organic acid found in animal products that participates in cellular metabolic reactions,[385] through its conversion to **phosphocreatine (PCr)** via the enzyme **creatine kinase (CK).**[386] PCr is a high energy reserve that can regenerate ATP from its breakdown product ADP (adenosine diphosphate)) through the donation of a phosphate molecule.[387] The **CK/PCr system** has three separate energy-related functions:[388]

	CK/PCr Energy Functions
1.	Immediately available energy buffer
2.	Energy shuttle (transport) system
3.	Metabolic regulator

Maintenance of cell homeostasis depends upon mechanisms that adjust the ATP generation processes according to energy demand.[389] This requires that ATP is sent to its sites of use, whilst it breakdown product, **ADP,** is stored and recycled.[390] **The phosphocreatine system is fundamental in promoting rapid re-synthesis of ATP by creatine kinase.**[391] It is particularly important in situations of high metabolic demand - such as high-intensity physical exercise, where the rate of ATP use exceeds its capacity for generation by other metabolic pathways.[392]

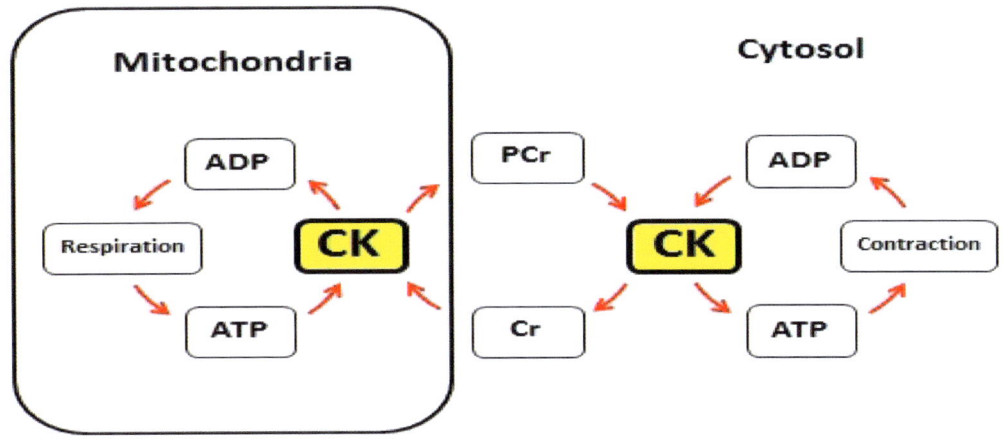

ATP = adenosine triphosphate; ADP = adenosine diphosphate; Cr = creatine; CK = creatine kinase; PCr = phosphocreatine

Since ATP production is in the interior of the mitochondria and the locations of use are in the cytosol, an overlapping mechanism of transfer is essential.[393] It is the CK/PCr system that acts as an energy shuttle which connects sites of ATP production (mitochondrial respiration) with sites of ATP utilisation (cell membrane ATPase enzymes).[394] The shuttle mechanism occurs via the co-expression of cytosolic specific CK with mitochondrial specific CK.[395] The energy producing and consuming terminals of the shuttle are connected via phosphocreatine and creatine, with no need for ATP or ADP to diffuse from the mitochondria to the sites of ATPases or backwards.[396] This allows for the build-up of a large cytosolic PCr pool - of up to 30 mM – using ATP predominantly from aerobic respiration or from glycolysis.[397] In the absence of creatine, high concentrations of ADP are needed for mitochondrial respiration; hence **creatine is a stimulator of mitochondrial respiration**[398]

Creatine supplementation has emerged as a safe nutritional supplement to strengthen cellular energetics.[399] Animal studies have shown that life-long creatine supplementation, even at a very high daily dosage, is of significant benefit for life quality of normal healthy mice;[400] whereas in humans, a change of lifestyle, together with creatine intake may prevent or delay the onset of health problems such as obesity, type-2 diabetes and metabolic syndrome.[401] Creatine is particularly important for normal brain function[402] because during times of brain activity, brain phosphocreatine decreases rapidly to maintain constant ATP levels.[403] Supplementation can improve mood and cognitive function during times of low energy or fatigue,[404] and is especially useful when performing demanding or complex cognitive tasks.[405] Daily requirements for creatine are approximately **2-4 g/day**,[406] of which around 0.25-1.0 g/day is obtained from a typical omnivorous diet.[407] Long-term supplementation at 4 g/day has been shown to be safe.[408]

Creatine dosage	• 2-4 g/day

Omega-3 Fats

Omega-3 fatty acids play a role in energy regulation through their ability to activate PPARs and induce AMPK (the fuel sensing and energy balancing enzyme), together with regulating cell membrane fluidity and function.[409] Inducement of AMPK increases fat breakdown and reduces fat storage.[410] Omega-3 deficiency, however, produces a metabolic shift in favour of fat and cholesterol synthesis at the expense of fat breakdown,[411] and contributes to the development of insulin resistance, metabolic syndrome and NAFLD.[412] Metabolic disturbances in the brain are now linked to metabolic syndrome - which impact on mood and cognitive function - and could explain why omega-3 supplementation can help with mood and emotional disorders.[413] Such disturbances may be a result of inflammation (a consequence of metabolic syndrome) in the hypothalamus, which disrupts metabolic control of energy balance, leading to insulin resistance, obesity and cardiovascular disease.[414]

Supplementation of omega-3 fats in the form of fish oil can maintain proper insulin signalling in the brain, improve NAFLD and decrease the risk of metabolic syndrome.[415] A reduction in some markers of metabolic syndrome can occur with supplementation at approximately **1 g/day**,[416],[417] whilst at the level of 3 g/day (1.086 g EPA, 0.72g DHA) it can improve body composition, especially reduced abdominal fat mass, in obese individuals.[418] Fish oil is the preferred source because the active substances - **EPA-(eicosapentaenoic acid)** and **DHA (docosahexaenoic acid)** – are already preformed; whereas vegetarian sources such as linseed oil contain the precursor alpha-linolenic acid, which needs to be enzymatically converted to EPA and DHA. This conversion rate is very low, especially for DHA, with around 30% in total for women and 16%

for men.[419] The only vegetarian source that contains EPA and DHA preformed, albeit not as high, is from algae. So for vegetarians, the best supplement would be algal supplements.

Omega-3 dosage
- Total = 1 -3g/day
- EPA = 500 - 1,000 mg/day
- DHA = 375 - 750 mg/day

Summary

HEALTH FOUNDATION SUPPLEMENTS

	Product	Function	Dosage
1.	**Multi-Vitamin & Mineral**	Broad spectrum vitamin and mineral support. Fills nutritional gaps.	Optimum multi
2.	**Probiotics**	Improve gut barrier function, energy absorption, gut motility, appetite regulation, glucose and lipid metabolism, and liver fat storage.	10 billion p/day *(lactobacillus & bifidobacteria)*
3.	**Milk Thistle (Silymarin)**	Improves liver function - central to metabolic energy homeostasis and detoxification.	140 mg/day
4.	**Vitamin C**	Antioxidant - protects cells from free radical damage. Helps regulate lipid metabolism.	1,000 mg/day

ENERGY SPECIFIC SUPPLEMENTS

	Product	Function	Dosage
1.	**Magnesium**	Central role in energy metabolism and ATP production. Bound to ATP molecule. Co-factor	200-450 mg/day

		in over 300 metabolic reactions.	
2.	**Calcium**	Regulates enzymes involved in ATP production. Central to muscle function.	160-360 mg/day
3.	**B-Vitamins**	Co-factors in mitochondrial energy production.	**Most = 50 mg/day** **Folic Acid = 400 mcg** **B12/Biotin = 50 mcg**
4.	**Alpha Lipoic Acid**	Co-factor in glucose breakdown. Activates fuel sensing enzyme and metabolism clock genes. Works synergistically with CoQ10.	600 mg/day
5.	**L-Carnitine**	Transports fats into the mitochondria for breakdown. Carnitine enzyme in brain acts as a nutrient sensing signalling mechanism that regulates feeding.	3 g/day *(Acetyl-L-Carnitine)*
6.	**CoQ10**	Critical co-factor in final part of ATP production. Activates fuel sensing enzyme & metabolism clock genes. Works synergistically with ALA.	100-300 mg/day
7.	**Creatine**	Stimulates mitochondrial ATP production. High energy reserve that regenerates ATP at rapid rates over short periods where high metabolic demand.	2-4 g/day
8.	**Omega 3 Fats**	Activates enzyme fuel sensor and metabolism clock genes. Regulates cell membrane function.	1-3 g/day *EPA = 500-1,000 mg* *DHA = 373-750 mg*

Chapter 13: Exercise

Health Consequences of Inactivity

The rising incidence of health conditions related to physical inactivity and their links to endocrine dysfunction continue to challenge worldwide health care programmes.[420] Exercise is now widely recognised as an effective counter-measure to the development of metabolic diseases such as obesity, diabetes and cardiovascular disease.[421] Repeated exercise has been shown to improve insulin sensitivity,[422] increase fat breakdown[423] and maintain muscle metabolic capacity with ageing.[424] New evidence suggests that both skeletal muscle and adipose tissue function as integrated endocrine organs in response to exercise.[425]

The Energy Systems

There are three systems in the body that create ATP energy. They work simultaneously but the contribution from each depends upon the type of exercise, as well as its intensity and duration:

System	Type	Energy Duration
Sprint	ATP-CP	Provides energy for a **7-10 second sprint** without oxygen. Creatine phosphate (CP) is the high energy molecule that rapidly regenerates ADP back to ATP through the release of its phosphate molecule. Muscle CP storage is limited, so it is used up quickly.
High Power	Anaerobic	Provides energy for a **90 second power burst** without oxygen. Fast breakdown of glucose but only provides 2 molecules of ATP - along with lactic acid (a waste product), which can cause muscle fatigue.
Endurance	Aerobic	Provides energy for **periods longer than 90 seconds** – the length of time depends upon how fit you are. It is a much slower system that requires oxygen but provides 38 molecules of ATP from glucose breakdown. It can also use fat to produce ATP.

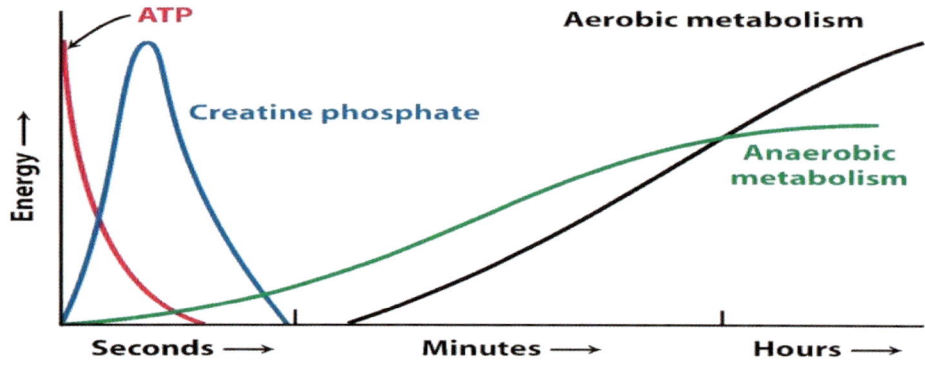

Source: Biochem 7th Ed, 2012. M H Freeman & Co

During exercise, skeletal muscle can increase its resting energy turnover by 1,000 times to meet the demands of exercise.[426] Because ATP is not stored in large quantities, ATP is re-synthesised from ADP at a rate to meet the metabolic demands of the cell; with muscle cell contraction initiating both ATP breakdown and re-synthesis.[427] Muscle phosphocreatine (PCr) is the most immediate substrate for ATP re-synthesis and can sustain a maximum ATP turnover rate for about 7-10 seconds.[428] Although muscles can also utilise carbohydrates and fat, the rates at which these can re-synthesis ATP is lower, although their capacity is greater. So, there is a trade-off between the power to produce ATP and the capacity for ATP production.[429] Hence, increasing exercise duration is achieved at the expense of the rate of ATP turnover.

Energy Fuel

Carbohydrates, fats and proteins are the three main energy fuels. The preferred energy fuel for muscles is glucose, especially as exercise intensity increases. However, the type of fuel used depends upon both exercise intensity and duration:[430]

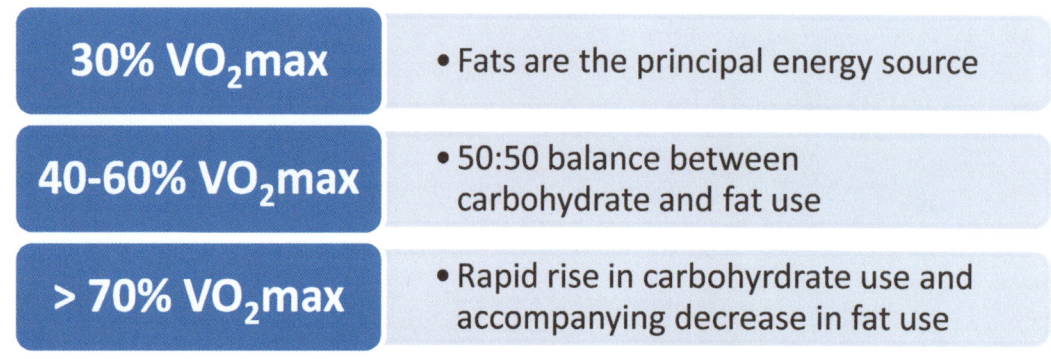

VO_2max = maximum oxygen volume uptake

During low-intensity exercise (which uses < 300 kcal/hr), you use a greater proportion of fat, a smaller proportion of glucose and fewer calories. As exercise intensity increases, your body will gradually use less fat, more glucose and more calories. Therefore, **most of the fuel during moderate and high intensity exercise (using > 500 kcal/hr) will come from glucose**. If you continue to exercise aerobically for a longer period, your body will gradually use more fat and less glucose in an attempt to conserve the limited glucose stores. The fitter you are, the more efficiently your muscles use fat and the longer you can work out.

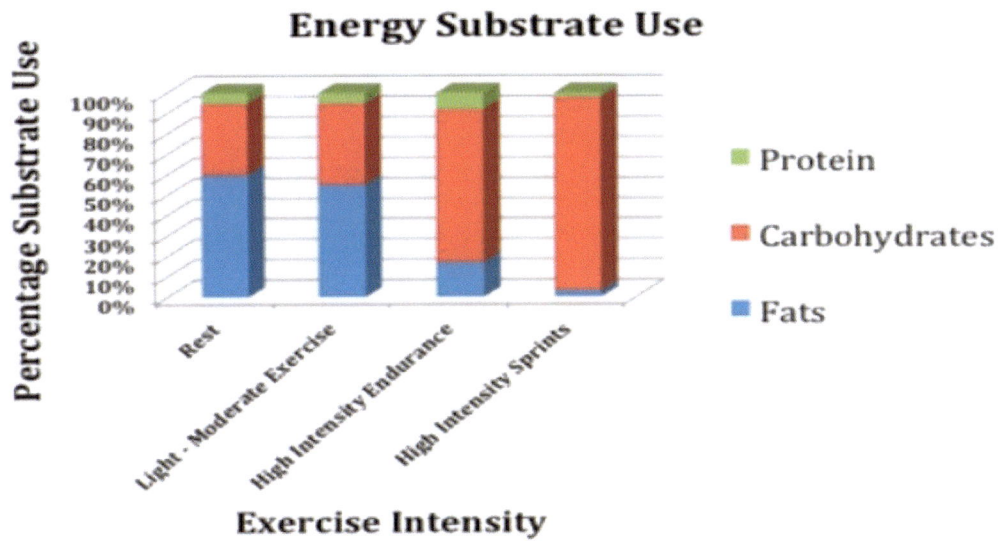

Source: www.kaizenactive.co.uk

Blood Glucose Maintenance

The maintenance of blood glucose during exercise represents a significant challenge because the rate of muscle glucose uptake increases several fold.[431] The principle organ for regulating blood glucose is the liver, which increases hepatic glucose production through glycogen breakdown. Glucose is stored as glycogen in the muscles as well as the liver; however, the body can only store a limited amount – equating to around 450 g for a 70 kg person – and so will also need to use fat stored in adipose tissue as an additional energy source.[432] Hence, a corresponding rise in the adrenal hormones *adrenaline* and *nor-adrenaline* (which increase fat release from adipose tissue) coincides with an increase in liver glucose output.[433]

At moderate to high intensity exercise (60-80% VO$_2$max), *cortisol* is also stimulated from the adrenals, with levels remaining high post-exercise.[434] Cortisol raises blood glucose levels through **gluconeogenesis** – the generation of glucose from non-carbohydrate sources, such as protein and glycerol. The peak breakdown of fatty acids occurs at approximately 65% VO_2max.[435] During the latter stages of prolonged moderate intensity exercise, there is a shift in fuel utilisation from carbohydrate to fatty acids; partly because of carbohydrate depletion but also due to the rise of adrenaline and fatty acids.[436]

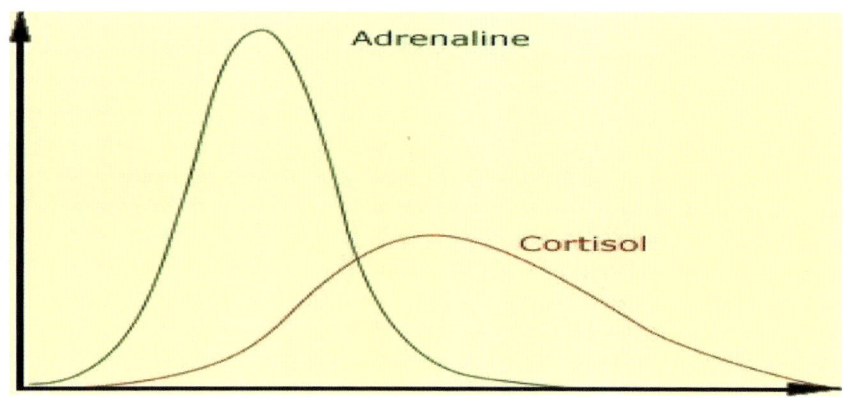

Source: www.hopestreetcentre.co.uk

Exercise and Fatigue

Carbohydrates are the most important nutrient for exercise because they are the ONLY fuel that can power intense exercise for prolonged periods. Even during anaerobic exercise when fatigue is initially due to CP depletion and the build-up of lactic acid, repeated bouts of this activity will also result in glycogen depletion. Yet, carbohydrate stores in the form of glycogen are very limited. If you do not re-stock your glycogen stores sufficiently, then you will run out of fuel after a few days of exercise or you will find that you feel fatigued.

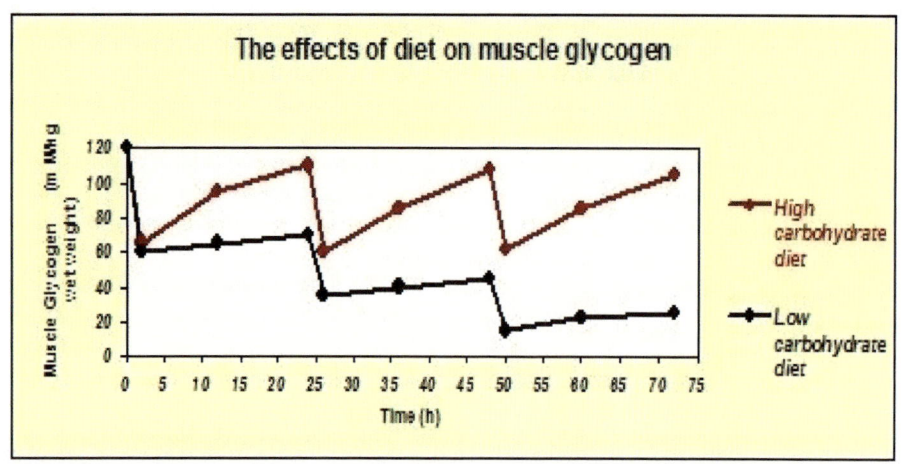

Costill, D.L., Miller, J.M. Nutrition for endurance sport: Carbohydrate and fluid balance. Int. J. Sports. Med. 1:2-14, 1980.

This is why embarking upon a low-carbohydrate diet, alongside an exercise programme can be counter-productive as you will not have sufficient fuel to power your exercise and you will soon start to feel tired. Therefore, if you want to exercise longer and harder, then you need to start off each exercise session by having a full tank of glucose and that's by eating a diet rich in carbohydrates. Just make sure that you are filling your tank with the healthy carbohydrates and not the energy-sapping bad ones.

Stress and Adrenal Fatigue

There is a direct link between exercise and adrenal fatigue.[437] Exercise itself is a stressor that leads to activation of the adrenal hormones in order to provide fuel for energy. Hence, if you exercise too much or too intensively when already under stress, you can exceed your capacity to cope, leading to adrenal insufficiency.[438] Adrenal insufficiency is the inability of the adrenal glands to produce a normal quantity of hormones (adrenaline, nor-adrenaline and cortisol).[439] This can have the effect of actually reducing your energy levels leading to fatigue. Adrenal insufficiency is now well recognised amongst athletes who over-train and are under other stresses – it's the total amount of the stressors that counts – leading to a condition called *Overtraining Syndrome (OS);* which can be described as "burnout" or chronic fatigue.[440] *Burnout* is the body's protection mechanism against unnecessary and potentially dangerous long-term stress as it reduces your energy levels and causes you to rest and conserve energy.[441]

There are striking similarities in the symptoms of chronic fatigue syndrome and in OS,[442] including the reduced capacity to exercise, which is primarily due to adrenal insufficiency.[443] This is hardly surprising when you consider that the mechanisms of energy production require adrenal hormones to stimulate the release and breakdown of energy stores to provide the fuel for exercise. So, although exercise is effective against the development of metabolic disorders, if you are under a lot of stress you will need to ensure that your exercise is gentle and moderate in the first instance and not excessive or too intense.

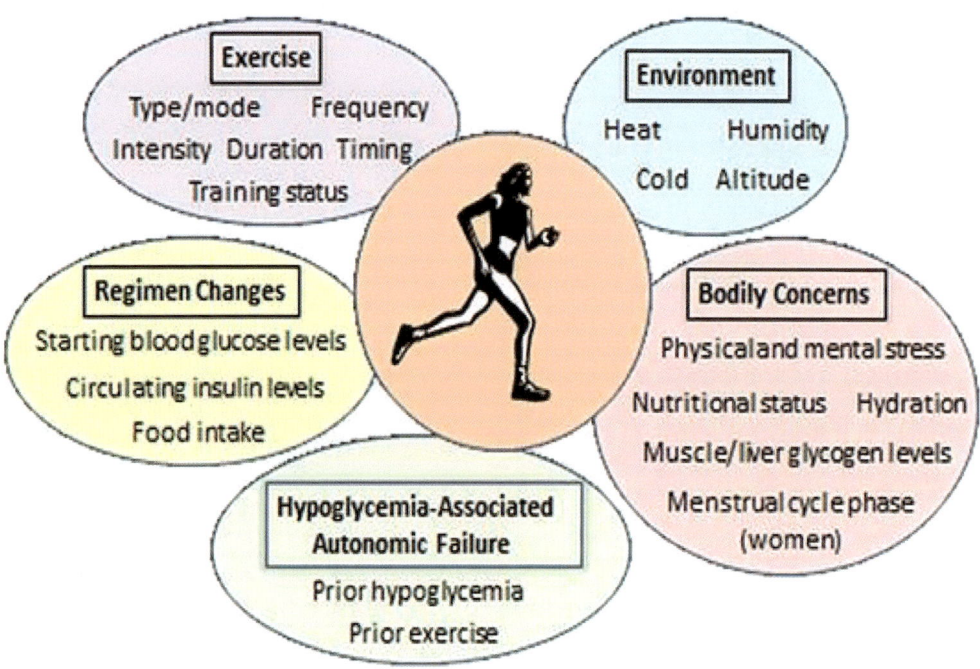

Source: www.diabetesmotion.com

Exercise Recommendations

For metabolic disorders, current physical activity guidelines recommend a ***daily minimum of 30 minutes of moderate-intensity physical activity***; with a preference for 60 minutes of moderate-intensity brisk walking to be supplemented by other activities.[444] These can include multiple short (10-15 minutes) bouts of activity (walking breaks at work, gardening, housework); using simple exercise equipment (e.g. treadmills); jogging; swimming; biking; golfing; team sports; and resistance training. A combination of aerobic and resistance exercise is best; however, any type of physical activity is encouraged and will provide benefit.

General Exercise Recommendations	
Daily Minimum	**30 minutes** of moderate-intensity physical exercise.
Ideal Daily Requirements	**60 minutes** of moderate-intensity exercise, plus other activities.
Types of Exercise	Combination of aerobic and resistance exercise.

If you have been sedentary for some time, lifestyle activity should be increased slowly in intensity and duration (by 5 minutes/session/week), starting from a low-intensity exercise to avoid excessive fatigue, muscle pain, strains or injuries.[445] You can start with short bouts (10 minutes each) rather than one long session to accumulate more minutes of exercise; or you could try using a pedometer and add 500 steps at 3-day intervals to a target value of 10,000-12,000 steps/day.[446]

Exercise Recommendations for the Sedentary	
Daily Minimum	**10-30 minutes** of low-intensity physical exercise.
Exercise Duration	**Start with 10 minutes per day** and then each week increase the duration by 5 minutes up to the daily minimum of 30 minutes or the ideal of 60 minutes. Alternatively, split the bouts of activity into 10 minute sessions.
Types of Exercise	Low-intensity aerobic exercise.

The impact of exercise on insulin sensitivity is evident for 24-28 hours and disappears within five days.[447] Therefore, it is important to exercise for at least 30 minutes per day most days of the week[448] for a continued benefit of exercise on insulin action. Avoiding or reducing common leisure sedentary activities, such as watching TV and playing computer games, is also advised.

Chapter 14: Stimulants

Caffeine

Caffeine is a stimulant of the central nervous system (CNS) and is the most commonly used **psychoactive drug** in the world that is legal and unregulated.[449] It is also a known ergogenic aid that can enhance performance in high-intensity exercise.[450] In nature, it comes from the seeds, nuts or leaves of plants native to South America and is commercially now found in coffee, tea, energy drinks and chocolate. In North America, 90% of adults consume caffeine daily,[451] whilst it is estimated that the majority of the world's adult population consumes caffeine in sufficient doses to influence their behaviour on a daily basis.[452] A cup of coffee contains approximately 80-175 mg of caffeine, depending upon what seed (bean) is used and how it is prepared. It is generally recognised as safe because typically used doses are under 500 mg/day, whereas toxic doses can range from 3-10 g/day for an adult.[453]

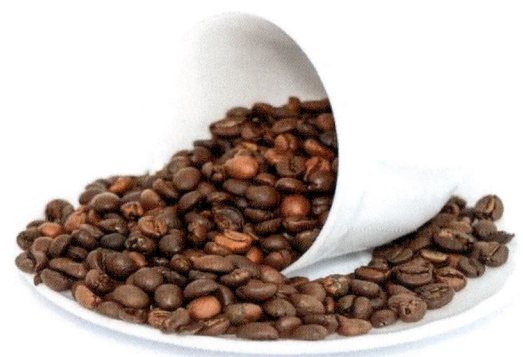

Source: www.pixabay.com

The most prominent mechanism of action of caffeine is to reversibly block the action of adenosine on its receptor and reduce adenosine transmission in the brain.[454] Adenosine forms part of the ATP (adenosine triphosphate) molecule involved in energy production. However, in the nervous system, ATP acts as a co-transmitter in extracellular signalling, where it is involved in neurotransmission (nerve message delivery).[455] Neurons (nerve cells) release ATP into the extracellular tissue,[456] where it is broken down to adenosine via ectoenzymes (enzymes outside of a cell).[457] In this way, adenosine exerts a broad spectrum of physiological and pathophysiological functions,[458] including modulating neurotransmission, immune regulation, vascular function and metabolic control.[459]

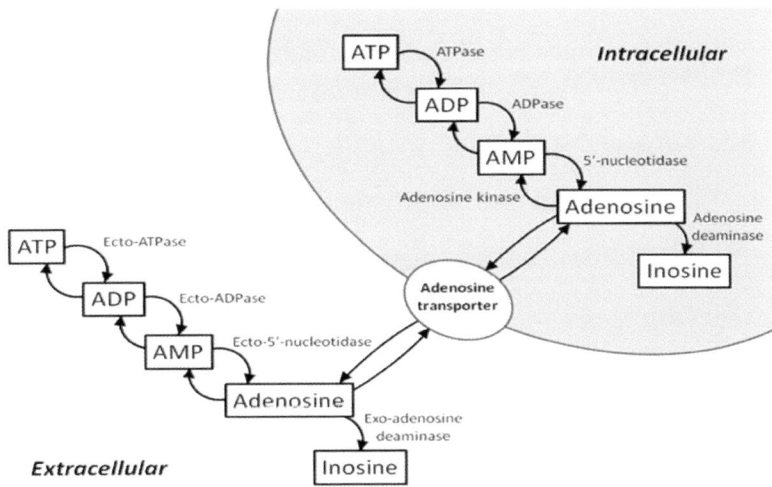

Source: www.journal.frontiersin.org

ATP-dependent adenosine signalling typically occurs during conditions that are associated with ATP release from intracellular stores,[460] such as when there is a demand for energy. Extracellular adenosine levels can rise in conditions of extreme physiology, such as strenuous exercise or at high altitude, where there are low oxygen levels.[461]

Caffeine blockage of the adenosine receptors prevents adenosine activation of nerve messages,[462] which enables caffeine to exert a wide range of effects. One of the primary actions of adenosine is to make you tired or sleepy; so by blocking the uptake of adenosine, caffeine will delay fatigue onset and make you more alert and energetic. In addition, this blockage also alters the production of most of the other major neurotransmitters including dopamine, acetylcholine, serotonin and nor-adrenaline; which in turn can improve your mood, increase your mental energy and muscular activity, suppress your appetite and relieve depression.[463]

Despite the potential benefits, taken in excess, caffeine can lead to adverse health effects. In particular, adverse cardiovascular effects have been found which include impaired blood vessel dilation, increased blood pressure,[464] arterial and aortic stiffness,[465] and myocardial infarction.[466] Ingestion of as little as 200 mg or more of caffeine can lead to tachycardia (fast heart rate) and arrhythmia (irregular heart beat).[467] Frequent consumption can also negatively impact cognition and memory;[468] whilst at doses of 300-400 mg can increase anxiety and tension.[469] Hallucinatory experiences can also occur with doses greater than 300 mg/day of coffee (approximately 7 cups);[470] whilst caffeine poisoning has recently been identified, with arrhythmias being the most common cause of caffeine-related death.[471]

Caffeine is generally well absorbed and achieves peak blood levels 15-45 minutes following ingestion.[472] However, the effects on the body are linked with individual metabolism and environmental factors.[473] Current knowledge suggests that a dose of 400 mg/day for healthy adults is not associated with adverse effects but it really does depend upon individual metabolism as well as lifestyle factors.[474] Also, the content of caffeine in many brands can vary widely, so 400 mg/day could range from between 2-5 cups, depending upon the brand. And, be aware that alcohol can prolong its action and contribute to its toxic effects.[475] The best advice is to **keep caffeine consumption to a minimum.**

Energy Drinks

The consumption of energy drinks has substantially increased during the past few decades, especially in Western and Asian countries.[476] Although manufacturers claim these drinks are beneficial in that they can boost energy, as well as physical and cognitive performance, there is insufficient scientific evidence to support these claims.[477] Conversely, energy drinks and their ingredients are potentially dangerous to many aspects of health and represent a global public health problem.[478] As a consequence, the American Institute of Medicine published a report in 2007 in respect of adolescents recommending that they restrict carbonated, fortified or flavoured waters, as well as the prohibition of energy drink use generally and caffeinated products in schools.[479]

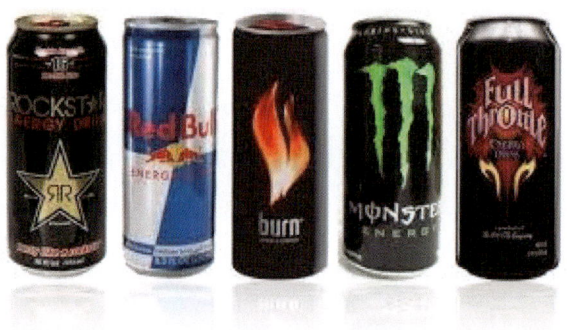

Source: www.themindunleashed.org

Energy drinks are fortified beverages with added dietary supplements. They differ from soft or sports drinks in that they contain higher levels of caffeine (which is their main ingredient), in addition to sugars and other dietary supplements.[480] Consumption of sugar-sweetened beverages – including energy drinks, soft drinks, fruit drinks and vitamin water drinks – is positively associated with overweight and obesity,[481] as well as an increased risk of diabetes mellitus and cardiovascular diseases.[482]

High caffeine consumption, whether through coffee or energy drink consumption, can lead to adverse health conditions. In recent years, several types of these high-caffeinated energy drinks have been linked to unexpected deaths in apparently healthy people - which has led to investigations by the US Food & Drug Administration (FDA) into the product safety.[483] The swift change in public perception of energy drinks from harmless mild stimulant to lethal, unregulated drug is unprecedented.[484] **The advice is very clear with regards to energy drinks – do not drink them.**

Alcohol

Athletes of ancient times used alcohol as an energy enhancer to improve performance, whilst the modern-day stressed adult of the 21st century will often use alcohol as an energy crutch to boost their flagging energy levels. The reality, however, is that the opposite is true – alcohol impedes energy production. Acute, chronic and even moderate ingestion of alcohol have been shown to elicit negative consequences.

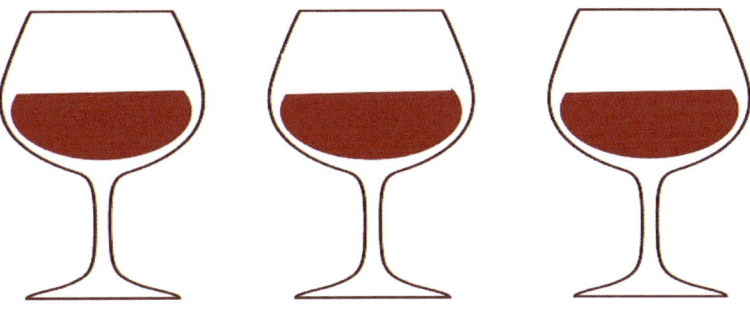

Source: www.pixabay.com

Alcohol is widely consumed in most parts of the world and has long been associated with various liver diseases accounting for about 4% of all deaths.[485] However, it may also be linked with metabolic disorders such as obesity, type-2 diabetes, and metabolic syndrome.[486] In the US, 50% of the adult population consumes alcohol on a regular basis,[487] whilst in the UK that rises to almost 80%.[488] Alcohol misuse is a leading cause of ill-health in the UK.[489]

The effects of alcohol are multiple since it targets many brain neurotransmitters in the central nervous system (CNS),[490] via increasing extracellular adenosine signalling.[491] In particular, it promotes a depressive effect in the CNS by inhibiting the release of **glutamate** *(the main excitatory neurotransmitter)*[492] and increasing **GABA** *(gamma-aminobutyric acid - the main inhibitory neurotransmitter)*.[493] Levels of **dopamine** are also increased in the reward pathway;[494] whilst an increase in **endorphins** provide a "high"; and increased **nor-adrenaline** and **adrenaline** provide stimulatory effects.[495] Like caffeine, alcohol alters adenosine neurotransmission; however, whereas caffeine stimulates the CNS, alcohol depresses it.[496]

Excessive chronic or binge (acute large doses) drinking can cause hepatic steatosis (abnormal retention of lipids), which can progress to more advanced forms of alcoholic liver disease (ALD), such as fibrosis and cirrhosis.[497] Hepatic steatosis is the earliest response to alcohol consumption and develops in 90% of heavy alcohol drinkers.[498] In simple cases it is usually asymptomatic, reversible and resolves after 4-6 weeks of abstinence.[499] With continuous alcohol intake, 20%-30% will develop alcoholic hepatitis and 16% will develop cirrhosis.[500] Alcoholic cirrhosis is irreversible and is among the top ten causes of death worldwide.[501]

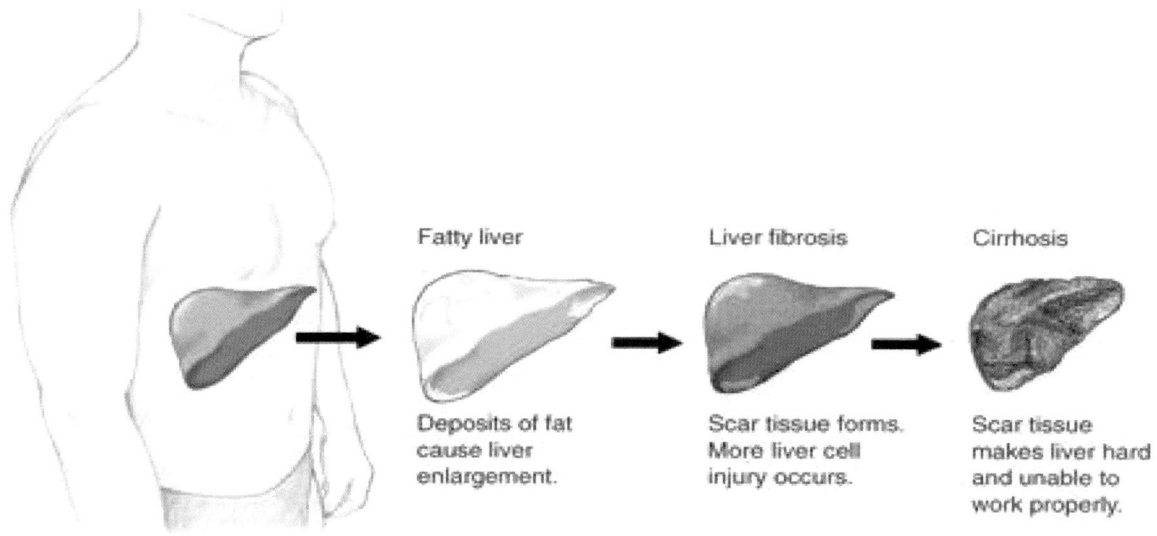

Source: www.healthtestingcenters.com

Approximately 90% of ingested alcohol is rapidly absorbed into the bloodstream from the stomach and small intestine, where it distributes into total body water.[502] On an empty stomach, peak blood levels occur about 30 minutes after ingestion.[503] However, because alcohol absorption occurs more quickly in the small intestine, food in the stomach slows down alcohol absorption as it delays gastric emptying - especially where the food has a high fat content.[504]

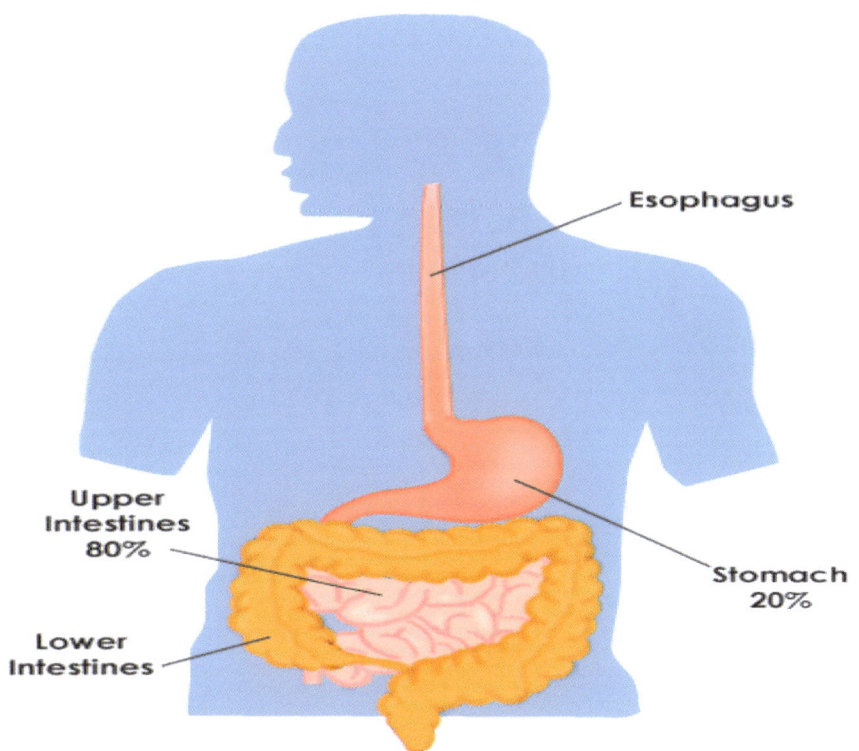

Source: www.science.howstuffworks.com

Alcohol metabolism occurs primarily in the liver (although a small amount is metabolised in the stomach) via three enzymes: **alcohol dehydrogenase (ADH), cytochrome P450 2E1 (CYP2E1)** and **catalase**; but it is ultimately metabolised inside the mitochondria via the Krebs cycle.[505] Metabolism occurs at a steady rate – typically between 15-20 mg/hour – irrespective of how much has been consumed.[506] However, this rate varies depending upon several factors including rates of absorption and metabolism, gender, body weight, percentage of body water, use of medications, the rate of drinking and concurrent food consumption.[507]

Inside the mitochondria, alcohol inhibits **PPARs** (the gene regulators of enzymes involved in glucose and lipid metabolism), which increases fatty acid synthesis and decreases fatty acid breakdown; thereby transforming the liver into a fat storage organ.[508] Chronic alcohol consumption can cause changes in mitochondrial structure and function, which are associated with the development of fatty liver[509] and impairment of hepatic energy metabolism.[510] Hence, the mitochondria play a major role in alcohol induced hepatic fat accumulation.[511] Because the liver is the main organ responsible for metabolising ingested alcohol, it is also the most susceptible to alcohol related injury.[512] Such injury can result from acetaldehyde toxicity (alcohol metabolite) or from gut endotoxins that have moved through the gut barrier as a result of alcohol disrupting the gut barrier function.[513]

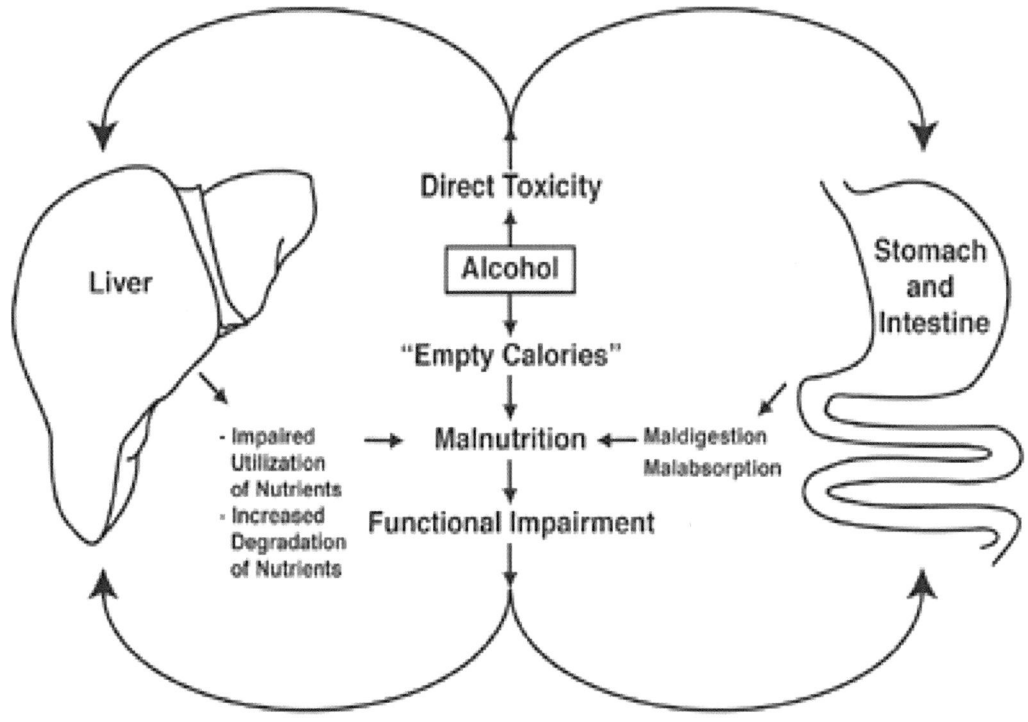

Source: www.mcieast.marines.mil

Alcohol-induced changes have a profound impact on the functioning of a wide-variety of organs and biological processes, which are dependent upon the central circadian clock synchronisation for proper function.[514] Such circadian disruption is a likely consequence of alcohol metabolism - acetaldehyde in particular - and the alcohol-induced change in intestinal barrier integrity.[515] Both these mechanisms induce systemic inflammation, which disrupts the circadian rhythmicity.[516] Rhythmic hormones such as cortisol and melatonin are significantly affected by this disruption,[517] whilst the immune system is negatively influenced leading to immune dysregulation.[518] This internal misalignment scenario has now been linked to weight gain, obesity and the metabolic syndrome.[519]

The negative consequences of alcohol consumption are very clear and are particularly detrimental to energy levels. With such a high percentage of the population regularly consuming alcohol, it is not surprising that alcohol and its related health conditions are on the rise. Concurrently arising with alcohol intake is circadian disruption, metabolic dysfunction and impaired energy production. If you want to improve your energy levels, then keep alcohol intake to a minimum or eliminate it altogether. If you do drink, then make sure you are well hydrated before drinking and do not drink on an empty stomach.

Key Points

Caffeine	• Restrict to 2 cups per day.
Energy Drinks	• Avoid entirely.
Alcohol	• Keep to a minimum. Ensure you are well-hydrated and do not drink on an empty stomach.

Chapter 15: Conclusion

Overview

We live in an environment that continually places demands upon us – both real and perceived. Our bodies need to be able to adapt to such demands. Physical events, psychological or anticipatory factors can cause us to diverge from a state of equilibrium. The body will always try to restore homeostasis through a series of complex physiologic and behavioural responses that aim to restore the challenged body to a state of equilibrium. Yet, this very process consumes energy stores and nutrients that can leave us nutrient and energy depleted. This is further compounded by an unhealthy diet, lack of exercise and lifestyle factors that further deplete energy stores. As a consequence, fatigue and energy-related disorders are approaching epidemic levels. Symptoms can be multiple and can affect the physical, emotional and mental levels. Wellbeing across the generations is being compromised by a lack of understanding of energy dynamics and what can be done to improve energy levels and ultimately health.

Energy Definitions

The statistics show that of those fatigue suffers who consult their doctors, 50% will remain undiagnosed by their doctor after one year with the condition. This leaves them with no explanation as to the reason for their condition and without a treatment plan to help them overcome their problem. These are shocking figures. By understanding energy dynamics and following the **Energy Programme Plan** you will be able to take back control and start on the road to revived and sustained energy levels. The first step in understanding energy dynamics is to become familiar with the basic energy terms:

Energy Definitions	
Energy	Cannot be created or destroyed but it can be converted from one form to another.
Energy Sources	Environmental energy from food and/or the atmosphere is converted into biological energy in the body.
Energy Fuel	Carbohydrates, fats and proteins (in that order of priority) fuel

	metabolic reactions. **Carbohydrates are the main fuel.**
Energy Currency	**ATP** molecule produced in the mitochondria. Needs to be recycled constantly as it cannot store long-term energy.
Energy Unit	Expressed as a **calorie.** Relates to the energy needed to increase the temperature of 1 kg of water by 1°C.
Metabolism	Biological energy production occurs through a series of chemical reactions within the cells.
Cellular Respiration	Chemical mechanism inside of the cells that transfers energy from food into ATP energy.
Metabolic Regulator	**Glucose** – its concentration in the blood acts as the main control for insulin (which directs glucose to cells for energy or storage).
Metabolic Pathways	3 pathways – (1) cellular energy production; (2) fat storage; (3) heat dissipation. Hormonal, neural and metabolic signals control flow.
Energy Homeostasis	Balances energy intake with energy output, energy storage, activity and heat loss.
Energy Disruption	Disruption to the inter-linked nutritional, chemical, hormone and neurotransmitter messages involved in energy transfer.

Energy Dynamics

Energy dynamics is all about the mechanisms of energy production, utilisation and storage. It is a highly regulated system that is designed to promote energy supply to fuel your metabolic processes and sustain your survival. Potential energy from food is converted into biological ATP energy at the cellular level in the mitochondria (the energy batteries of the cells). This cellular energy production is termed metabolism or cellular respiration. The main process is aerobic respiration, which requires oxygen, but in the absence of oxygen, energy is generated via anaerobic respiration which does not require oxygen.

Energy production is governed by a regular 24-hour circadian cycle driven by clock genes throughout the body. These clock genes are regulated by the master clock ('the pacemaker') in the SCN (suprachiasmatic nucleus) of the hypothalamus. The hypothalamus is the area of the brain that links the nervous system to the endocrine system, whilst the SCN synchronises internal biological process to external time cues (such as day and night). Signals from the SCN are turned into hormonal signals via the hypothalamus in the form of the hormones melatonin (sleep hormone) and cortisol (stress hormone), which are the principal hormone clock messengers.

Specific hormones initiate fuel delivery to the cells and control the rate of energy production. Insulin and glucagon, which work together but in opposing ways, are the main regulators of fuel delivery. Insulin lowers blood glucose levels by removing glucose from the blood and delivering it to the cells for energy or storage. Conversely, glucagon raises blood glucose levels when levels fall too low by breaking down glycogen (stored glucose) in the liver and muscles. The energy back-up system involves the stress response mechanism of the adrenal hormones adrenaline, nor-adrenaline and cortisol. Together, these mobilise stored energy by triggering glucagon secretion, lipolysis (fat breakdown) and gluconeogenesis (glucose generation from proteins and other non-carbohydrate sources). Finally, the thyroid hormones control how quickly energy is produced by altering the rate of mitochondrial ATP production.

A central neural circuitry integrates sensory information (such as satiety or hunger) from the hypothalamus, along with input from the motivational system (such as food preferences) in the cortico-limbic system of the brain. Together, these provide information on energy deficit and specific food preferences (based on earlier food experiences that have previously generated a reward or gratification feeling). This sensory information is integrated, along with hormonal and energy substrate signals, in the ARC (arcuate nucleus) of the hypothalamus, which allows the brain to promote or limit food intake to regulate energy balance. The ARC is the crucial regulator of whole-body energy homeostasis that can be likened to *Mission Control*.

Energy Disruption

The complex nature of our highly regulated metabolism means that signal disturbances can occur at many levels. Energy dynamics involve inter-linked signals from nutritional, chemical, hormonal and neurotransmitter messages that need to be integrated together to provide the full message. Incomplete messages can distort the true picture. It is necessary to look at the main potential points of disturbance to identify where along the line your signals are being distorted.

Food is a good starting point, as food is your potential energy source that will be turned into biological ATP energy to power your body. The fast-food, processed convenience diet of today is markedly different from the historical low-energy density diet that the human gut was adapted to over several millennia. This has a major impact on the gastrointestinal system, which is the body's interface with contents from the external environment, and provides the initial feedback to the brain as to those contents that will result in a perception of hunger or satiety.

It is the gut that regulates appetite and delivery of nutrients to the blood by controlling food motility and absorption through a combination of nutrient, neural and hormonal messages. Diet is one of the most pivotal factors in the development of the gut microflora, which play an important role in stimulating the appetite-suppressing gut hormone signalling pathway to reduce food intake. However, the high consumption of fat and a low intake of fibre, fruit, vegetables and meat of today's diet are associated with a decreased microbial diversity. This has the effect of increasing GI tract transit time and absorption and reducing the appetite suppressing signals leading to excess consumption.

Integral to energy demand is stress of any kind, which is now so pervasive in today's society that it can often lay at the heart of energy related disorders. The stress mechanism, which invokes the adrenal hormones, is essential to our survival as it provides a critical back-up energy system in times of need by re-directing energy resources to the brain and the muscles for 'fight or flight'. This allows us to have amazing powers of speed and strength at times of crisis – essential to our ancestors escaping or fighting tigers but not so essential to emotional or perceived stress, which nevertheless provokes the same response. Chronic, prolonged stress without resolution can significantly disrupt metabolic pathways through over-stimulation of the adrenal hormones. Cortisol, in particular, can be especially damaging as it can shift metabolism from being anabolic (growth enhancing) to catabolic (breaking down); resulting in a redistribution of fat to central deposition, increased size and number of fat cells, decreased energy expenditure, disturbed gut flora, diminished satiety signals and an enhanced consumption of high fat foods.

Constant stimulation of any hormone ultimately leads to under-production as the raw materials required for production become scarcer. Unresolved stress will ultimately lead to an under-production of cortisol. Because cortisol is also the main anti-inflammatory of the body, when its production becomes blunted, it leads to increased inflammation as stress itself elicits inflammatory mediators. Inflammation is a normal immune response to injury or damage but if left uncontrolled, then it becomes damaging. This increased inflammation induces a re-allocation of energy directed towards the activated immune system, which is equivalent to that required by the brain and muscles. It also induces a rapid increase in thyroid hormone production (to increase energy production) followed by a rapid down-regulation of thyroid hormone production.

The involvement of the thyroid hormones goes hand-in-hand with their role in increasing the rate of cellular energy production. In this way, the increased ATP production can help to meet the energy demands brought on by the stressor. This is why increased cortisol secretion, which is all about re-direction of energy stores at times of energy need, always leads to altered thyroid hormone production and hence altered metabolism. Over-stimulation of cortisol, however, results in decreased thyroid gland stimulation and decreased conversion of the thyroid prohormone T_4 (thyroxine) to the active form T_3 (tri-iodothyronine), whilst at the same time increasing the conversion of T_4 to the inactive form rT_3. The effects of rT_3 are to slow metabolism and reduce cellular energy production by blocking but not activating the hormone receptors. In this way, it acts as a protective feedback mechanism to prevent over-stimulation of the mitochondria to produce ATP, which would otherwise be damaging to the cells.

The mitochondria are the cellular batteries of the body producing ATP energy. In response to changes in energy demand, the mitochondria adjust the rate and amount of ATP production. Because these organelles play a key role in energy production, their structure changes continuously between fusion (joining together) and fission (splitting of damaged material) in a sequentially repeating cycle. These structural changes allow them to adapt to different energy demands, whilst also enabling them to remove damaged material to effect repairs. Stress, cellular injury, nutrient excess, high fat diet and environmental toxins can shift the mitochondrial dynamics to fission, resulting in fragmentation, mitochondrial damage, excess generation of free radicals, oxidative stress and ultimately cell death. Such changes will impact severely on energy production leading to fatigue conditions.

The Energy Programme Plan in a Nutshell

Understanding how the body works is half the battle when it comes to implementing practical steps designed to enhance the natural energy dynamics. Following a specific programme plan becomes much easier when you know why you are doing what you are doing. The **Energy Programme Plan** is designed as a lifestyle plan that you gradually incorporate into your daily life so that ultimately it becomes your lifestyle rather than a short-term energy-boost plan. We all find change difficult and trying to introduce too much change at once can result in failure as we become overwhelmed. This Plan is about implementing a series of progressive steps within your own timeframe. Each change you make counts and will take you closer to the sustained energy that you desire. How much you choose to implement is entirely up to you.

Step	Key Features	Action
1. **Hydration**	Insufficient or ineffective hydration manifests as tiredness or hunger. Effective hydration = water + sodium	**Drink 1.5 L water p/d. Include salt when dehydrated.**
2. **Sleep**	Sleep restriction or disturbance disrupts metabolism. Both are governed by the master circadian clock. Jetlag/ shift work disrupts master clock signals. Light is the key factor in re-setting the biological clock.	**Follow sleeping tips in Chpt. 8 to set your optimal sleep schedule.**
3. **Stress Management**	Stress is a major contributor to energy disruption. It is your response to stress that matters not the size. Managing stress = taking charge of your thoughts emotions, schedule and the way that you deal with problems. Healthy coping strategies require change. Change = change your	**Identify your sources of stress. Employ the stress management strategies in Chpt. 9 to instigate change.**

		situation or change your reaction.	
4.	**Diet**	Healthy eating = developing a life-long eating plan. Incorporate small, manageable changes rather than one big drastic change. Key aspects = moderation and balance. Establish a regular daily eating pattern. Avoid sugar overload and know your food groups.	**Plan your diet around fibre-rich vegetables, fruit, wholegrains, lean proteins and good fats. Follow the advice in Chpt. 10.**
5.	**Supplements**	Food now contains 75% fewer micronutrients because of modern farming. Stress, aging and ubiquitous environmental toxins create a greater need for additional nutrients. Scientific evidence overwhelmingly supports supplement use. Health Foundation supplements will support general health and metabolism. Specific cellular energy supplements can be used to cope with increased metabolic demand or to quickly raise energy levels before tackling the basics.	**No requirement to take supplements. Choose according to your needs and see what works for you.**
6.	**Exercise**	Effective counter-measure against metabolic diseases. Glucose is the preferred energy fuel but the type of fuel used depends upon both exercise intensity and duration. Exercise stimulates the adrenal hormones to provide energy, so if under stress ensure your exercise is gentle and moderate.	**30-60 minutes of moderate-intensity exercise per day. Combine aerobic and resistance exercise. Eat carbohydrates before and after.**
7.	**Stimulants**	**Caffeine** – legal unregulated drug that stimulates the CNS. It blocks tiredness nerve messages during energy demand to delay fatigue and keep you alert. Toxic at high doses. Excess leads to adverse health conditions. **Energy Drinks** – insufficient scientific evidence to	**Caffeine – restrict to 2 cups per day.** **Energy Drinks – avoid**

support energy boost claims. High caffeine and sugar content. Contents found to be very dangerous to health.	**completely.**
Alcohol – significantly disrupts energy production. It also depresses the CNS, disrupts gut barrier function and the circadian rhythm, and causes metabolic dysfunction and liver disease. Prolongs the action of caffeine and contributes to its toxic effects.	**Alcohol – keep to a minimum. Ensure well hydrated before drinking and do not drink on an empty stomach.**

Final Thought

Current scientific understanding of the highly complex metabolic regulatory pathways is painting a much clearer picture of energy dynamics. The need to understand the physiological basis of metabolism is becoming increasingly important with the growing rise in energy-related disorders. This book gives you an overview of the current literature on energy dynamics and provides a practical plan based on how your body works, that will allow you to implement steps in your own lives to achieve your optimal energy levels.

About the Author

Jan Clementson

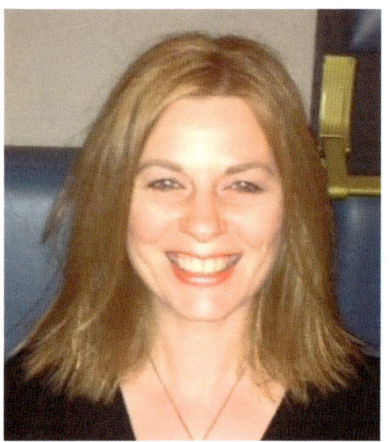

Jan is a UK qualified Nutritional Therapist who holds a first-class honours degree in Nutritional Medicine from the University of West London. She is a member of BANT (British Association for Applied Nutrition and Nutritional Therapy) and is registered with CNHC (The Complementary and Natural Healthcare Council). Her specialist area of interest is in metabolism, which encompasses energy, stress, weight control and sports nutrition. She is very passionate about health education and believes that understanding how the body works is the key to health. Previously, she has worked as lecturer in Biomedicine (anatomy, physiology and pathology) for London CNM (College of Naturopathic Medicine); a Clinical Nutrition Advisor for BioCare Ltd (a professional nutritional supplement company); as well as conducting individual nutritional consultancy work. Currently, she is in the process of setting up a Nutritional Therapy Practice in London.

Jan is British and grew up in Carlisle, Cumbria before moving to Leeds, New York, London, Birmingham and then back to London. She comes from a sporting background, specialising in track athletics and competed for her local running club, Border Harriers, for over 10 years. It was through her sporting background that she developed a keen interest in health and fitness but it was ultimately her life-long dairy intolerance that led her to nutrition. She initially started her career in law working in the local Magistrates' Courts where she qualified as a solicitor and worked as an in-court Legal Advisor. However, her interest in health and wellbeing led her to The Random House Book Publishing Group. Working in their health, fitness and wellbeing division inspired her to return to university to study nutrition and pursue her passion for health.

**You can contact Jan at: theenergysolution@hotmail.com
or on Facebook at: https://www.facebook.com/TheEnergySolutionEbook**

References

[1] Spiegelman B M & Flier J S (2001). Obesity and the regulation of energy balance. *Cell*, 104(4): 531-543.

[2] Spiegelman B M & Flier J S (2001). Obesity and the regulation of energy balance. *Cell*, 104(4): 531-543.

[3] Kondepudi, D. (2008). *Introduction to Modern Thermodynamics.* Chichester, UK: Wiley.

[4] G. P. Talwar, L. M. Srivastavaby, ed. (2003). *Textbook Of Biochemistry and Human Biology* (3 ed.). p.472.

[5] Kondepudi, D. (2008). *Introduction to Modern Thermodynamics.* Chichester, UK: Wiley.

[6] Murphy KG & Bloom SR (2006). Gut hormones and the regulation of energy homeostasis. *Nature* **444** (7121): 854-9.

[7] Murphy KG & Bloom SR (2006). Gut hormones and the regulation of energy homeostasis. *Nature* **444** (7121): 854-9.

[8] Subramaniam S, Fahy E, Gupta S, Sud M, Byrnes RW, Cotter D, Dinasarapu AR and Maurya MR (2011). "Bioinformatics and Systems Biology of the Lipidome". *Chemical Reviews* **111** (10): 6452–6490.

[9] Mehta S (2013). Oxidation of Fatty Acids. http://pharmaxchange.info/press/2013/10/oxidation-of-fatty-acids/ [Accessed 06/07/14].

[10] Brasaemle DL (2007). "Thematic review series: adipocyte biology. The perilipin family of structural lipid droplet proteins: stabilization of lipid droplets and control of lipolysis". *J. Lipid Res* **48** (12): 2547–59.

[11] Mehta S (2013). Digestion of Fats (Triacylglycoerols). http://pharmaxchange.info/press/2013/10/digestion-of-fats-triacylglycerols/ [Accessed 08/07/14].

[12] Mehta S (2013). Oxidation of Fatty Acids. http://pharmaxchange.info/press/2013/10/oxidation-of-fatty-acids/ [Accessed 06/07/14].

[13] Bairoch A (2000). "The ENZYME database in 2000". *Nucleic Acids Research* **28** (1): 304–305.

[14] Radzicka A, Wolfenden R (1995). "A proficient enzyme". *Science* **267** (5194): 90–93.

[15] Voet D, Voet JG. (2004). *Biochemistry* Vol 1 3rd ed. Hoboken, NJ, USA: Wiley.

[16] Brosnan J (June 2003). "Interorgan amino acid transport and its regulation". *Journal of Nutrition* **133** (6 Suppl 1): 2068S–72S.

[17] Rich PR (2003). "The molecular machinery of Keilin's respiratory chain". *Biochem. Soc. Trans.* **31** (Pt 6): 1095–105.

[18] Mehta S (2013). Energetics of Cellular Respiration (Glucose Metabolism). http://pharmaxchange.info/press/2013/10/energetics-of-cellular-respiration-glucose-metabolism/. [Accessed 08/07/14]/

[19] Knowles JR (1980). "Enzyme-catalyzed phosphoryl transfer reactions". *Annu. Rev. Biochem.* **49**: 877–919.

[20] Rich PR (2003). "The molecular machinery of Keilin's respiratory chain". *Biochem. Soc. Trans.* **31** (Pt 6): 1095–105.

[21] Törnroth-Horsefield S, Neutze R (December 2008). "Opening and closing the metabolite gate". *Proc. Natl. Acad. Sci. U.S.A.* **105** (50): 19565–6.

[22] Kleiner, SM (February 1999). "Water: an essential but overlooked nutrient". *Journal of the American Dietetic Association* **99** (2): 200.

[23] Armstrong L (2007). Performing in Extreme Environments. USA, Champaign IL: Human Kinetics.

[24] Ashcroft F, Life Without Water in Life at the Extremes. Berkeley and Los Angeles, 2000, 134-138.

[25] Shirreffs SM, Merson SJ, Fraser SM, Archer DT (June 2004). "The effects of fluid restriction on hydration status and subjective feelings in man". *Br. J. Nutr.* **91** (6): 951–8.

[26] Kaneshiro, Neil K. "Dehydration". National Library of Medicine. [Accessed 25/07/14].

[27] Bean, Anita (2006). *The Complete Guide to Sports Nutrition*. A & C Black Publishers Ltd. pp.81–83.

[28] Kaneshiro, Neil K. "Dehydration". National Library of Medicine. [Accessed 25/07/14].

[29] Danaei G et al (2011). National, regional, and global trends in fasting plasma glucose and diabetes prevalence since 1980: systematic analysis of health examination surveys and epidemiological studies with 370 country-years and 2·7 million participants. *The Lancet,* **378** (9785): 31-40.

[30] Wild S, Roglic G, Green A, Sicree R, King H. Global prevalence of diabetes: estimates for the year 2000 and projections for 2030. *Diabetes Care* 2004; 27: 1047-53.

[31] WHO 2013. Diabetes Factsheet No 312. http://www.who.int/mediacentre/factsheets/fs312/en/. [Accessed 23/07/14].

[32] Budd M L (2004) *Low Blood Sugar*. USA: Sterling.

[33] Cryer, Philip E. (2001). "Hypoglycemia". In Jefferson L, Cherrington A, Goodman H, eds. for the American Physiological Society. *Handbook of Physiology; Section 7, The Endocrine System*. II. The endocrine pancreas and regulation of metabolism. New York: Oxford University Press

[34] Hypoglycemia." It can also be referred to as "sugar crash" or "glucose crash." National Diabetes Information Clearinghouse, October 2008. http://diabetes.niddk.nih.gov/dm/pubs/hypoglycemia

[35] Mayo Clinic (2015). Hypoglycaemia – tests and diagnosis. www.mayoclinic.org. [Accessed 12/04/15].

[36] Pasquali R, Vicennati V, Cacciari M, Pagotto (2006).. The hypothalamic-pituitary-adrenal axis activity in obesity and the metabolic syndrome. Ann N Y Acad Sci.;1083:111-28.

[37] Arnold E & Boggs K U (2007). *Interpersonal Relationships*. St Louis, Missouri, USA: Saunders-Elsevier.

[38] Compare *The Stress of Life*, Hans Selye, New York: McGraw-Hill, 1956.

[39] Viner, R. (1999) Putting Stress in Life: Hans Selye and the Making of Stress Theory. *Social Studies of Science*, 29(3): 391–410.

[40] Bergman A et al (2010). State of Science of Endocrine Disrupting Chemicals. WHO.

[41] Evengård B, Schacterle RS, Komaroff AL (Nov 1999). "Chronic fatigue syndrome: new insights and old ignorance". *Journal of Internal Medicine* **246** (5): 455–469.

[42] *Guideline 53: Chronic fatigue syndrome/myalgic encephalomyelitis (or encephalopathy)*. London: National Institute for Health and Clinical Excellence. 2007.

[43] Sanders P, Korf J (2008). "Neuroaetiology of chronic fatigue syndrome: an overview". *World J. Biol. Psychiatry* **9** (3): 165–71.

[44] Wyller VB (2007). "The chronic fatigue syndrome--an update". *Acta neurologica Scandinavica. Supplementum* **187**: 7–14.

[45] http://www.drmyhill.co.uk. [Accessed 31/07/14].

[46] Wyller VB (2007). "The chronic fatigue syndrome--an update". *Acta neurologica Scandinavica. Supplementum* **187**: 7–14.

[47] Horton-Salway M (2007). "The ME Bandwagon and other labels: constructing the genuine case in talk about a controversial illness". *Br J Soc Psychol* **46** (Pt 4): 895–914.

[48] APPGME.org.uk" (PDF). [Retrieved 2011-01-28].

[49] Cullen W, Kearney Y, Bury G. (2002). Prevalence of fatigue in general practice. *Ir J Med Sci*, ;171:10-2.

[50] Cornuz J, Guessous I, Favrat B. (2006). Fatigue: a practical approach to diagnosis in primary care. *CMAJ* 174:765-7.

[51] Lewis G, Wessely S. (1992). The epidemiology of fatigue: more questions than answers. *J Epidemiol Community Health*,46:92-7.

[52] Hilsabeck RC, Hassanein TI, Perry W. (2005) Biopsychosocial predictors of fatigue in chronic hepatitis C. *J Psychosom Res*;58:173-8.

[53] EMedicine Health. "Fatigue Exams and tests" . [Accessed 25/01/10].

[54] Nijrolder I, van der Windt D, de Vries H, van der Horst H (November 2009). "Diagnoses during follow-up of patients presenting with fatigue in primary care". *CMAJ* **181** (10): 683–7.

[55] Nijrolder I, van der Windt D, de Vries H, van der Horst H (November 2009). "Diagnoses during follow-up of patients presenting with fatigue in primary care". *CMAJ* **181** (10): 683–7.

[56] Murray, R. & , J. (2001)Maughan, Ron J.; Murray, Robert, eds. (2001). "Ch. 8: Formulating carbohydrate-electrolyte drinks for optimal efficacy". *Sports Drinks: Basic Science and Practical Aspects*. CRC Press. pp.197–224

[57] Hypoglycemia." It can also be referred to as "sugar crash" or "glucose crash." National Diabetes Information Clearinghouse, October 2008. http://diabetes.niddk.nih.gov/dm/pubs/hypoglycemia.

[58] Hypoglycemia." It can also be referred to as "sugar crash" or "glucose crash." National Diabetes Information Clearinghouse, October 2008. http://diabetes.niddk.nih.gov/dm/pubs/hypoglycemia.

[59] Diabetes and Hypoglycemia". Diabetes.co.uk. Retrieved 2012-03-10.

[60] www.nhs.co.uk. [Accessed 03/08/14].

[61] Alfredo A A et al (2009). Chronic fatigue syndrome: aetiology, diagnosis and treatment. *BMC Psychiatry*, 9 (Suppl 1): SI.

[62] Price JR, Mitchell E, Tidy E, Hunot V (2008).: **Cognitive 3 behaviour therapy for chronic fatigue syndrome in adults.** *Cochrane Database Syst Rev*:CD001027.

[63] Alfredo A A et al (2009). Chronic fatigue syndrome: aetiology, diagnosis and treatment. *BMC Psychiatry*, 9 (Suppl 1): SI.

[64] Van Houdenhove B, Pae CU, Luyten P (2010). "Chronic fatigue syndrome: is there a role for non-antidepressant pharmacotherapy?". *Expert opinion on pharmacotherapy* **11** (2): 215–23.

[65] Rimes KA, Chalder T (2005). "Treatments for chronic fatigue syndrome". *Occupational Medicine* **55** (1): 32–39.

[66] http://www.elmhurst.edu/~chm/vchembook/592energy.html. [Accessed 12/07/14].

[67] Chen L & Yang G (2014). PPARs integrate the mammalian clock and energy metabolism *PPAR Research*, Article ID 653017.

[68] G.Yang, G. Paschos, A.M. Curtis, E. S.Musiek, S. C.McLoughlin, and G. A. Fitzgerald (2013). "Knitting up the raveled sleave of care," *Science Translational Medicine*, 5 (212), Article ID 212rv3.

[69] Tsang A, Barclay J L & Oster H (2014). Interactions between endocrine and circadian systems. Review. *Journal of Molecular Endocrinology*, 52: R1-R16.

[70] Tsang A, Barclay J L & Oster H (2014). Interactions between endocrine and circadian systems. Review. *Journal of Molecular Endocrinology*, 52: R1-R16.

[71] "Biological clock human" by NoNameGYassineMrabetTalk fixed by Addicted04 - The work was done with Inkscape by YassineMrabet. Informations were provided from "The Body Clock Guide to Better Health" by Michael Smolensky and Lynne Lamberg; Henry Holt and Company, Publishers (2000). Landscape was sampled from Open Clip Art Library (Ryan, Public domain). Vitruvian Man and the clock were sampled from Image:P human body.svg (GNU licence) and Image:Nuvola apps clock.png, respectively.. Licensed under CC BY-SA 3.0 via Wikimedia Commons - http://commons.wikimedia.org/wiki/File:Biological_clock_human.svg#/media/File:Biological_clock_human.svg

[72] Tsang A, Barclay J L & Oster H (2014). Interactions between endocrine and circadian systems. Review. *Journal of Molecular Endocrinology*, 52: R1-R16.

[73] G.Yang, G. Paschos, A.M. Curtis, E. S.Musiek, S. C.McLoughlin, and G. A. Fitzgerald (2013). "Knitting up the ravelled sleave of care," *Science Translational Medicine*, 5 (212), Article ID 212rv3.

[74] E. Maury, K. M. Ramsey, and J. Bass (2010). "Circadian rhythms and metabolic syndrome: from experimental genetics to human disease," *Circulation Research*, 106(3), pp. 447–462, 2010.

[75] Berthoud H-R et al (2012). Neural and metabolic regulation of macronutrient intake and selection. *Proc Nutr Soc*, 71(3): 390-400.

[76] Hussain S S & Bloom S R (2013). The regulation of food intake by the gut-brain axis: implications for obesity. *Int Journal of Obesity*, 37:625-633.

[77] Berthoud HR. Homeostatic and non-homeostatic pathways involved in the control of food intake and energy balance. Obesity (Silver Spring) 2006; 14(Suppl 5):197S–200S.

[78] Berthoud HR, Morrison C (2008) The brain, appetite, and obesity. *Annu Rev Psychol*, 59:55–92.

[79] Berthoud H-R et al (2012). Neural and metabolic regulation of macronutrient intake and selection. *Proc Nutr Soc*, 71(3): 390-400.

[80] Benoit SC, Davis JF, Davidson T (2010). Learned and cognitive controls of food intake. *Brain Res*, 1350:71–76

[81] Berthoud H-R et al (2012). Neural and metabolic regulation of macronutrient intake and selection. *Proc Nutr Soc*, 71(3): 390-400.

[82] Jezova D, Duncko R, Lassanova M, Kriska M, Moncek F (2002) . Reduction of rise in blood pressure and cortisol release during stress by ginkgo biloba extract (EGB 761) in healthy volunteers. J Physiol Pharmacol. 53(3):337-48.

[83] Iwen A et al (2013). Thyroid hormones and the metabolic syndrome. *Eur Thyroid J*, 2: 83-92.

[84] Gibbs J C et a (2011)l. The association of a high drive for thinness with energy deficiency and severe menstrual disturbances: confirmation in a large population of exercising women . Int J Sport Nut Exerc Metab, 21(4): 280-90.

[85] 1Golden SH, Robinson KA, Saldanha I, Anton B, Ladenson PW (2009). Prevalence and incidence of endocrine and metabolic disorders in the United States: a comprehensive review. *Journal of Clinical Endocrinology & Metabolism*. ;94(6):1853–1878.

[86] Amercian Thyroid Association. http://www.thyroid.org/media-main/about-hypothyroidism/. [Accessed 25/09/14].

[87] Thyroid UK. http://www.thyroiduk.org.uk/tuk/About_Us/study-report-5.01.12.html. [Accessed 25/09/14].

[88] International Diabetes Federation. Definition of the Metabolic Syndrome. http://www.idf.org/metabolic-syndrome. [Accessed 25/09/14].

[89] Zhang W, Cline M A & Gilber E R (2014). Hypothalams-adipose tissue crosstalk: neuropeptide Y and the regulation of energy metabolism. *Nutrition & Metabolism*, 11:27.

[90] Coll A P, Farooqui I S, O'Rahilly S (2007). The hormonal control of food intake. *Cell*, 29:251-262.

[91] Hussain S S & Bloom S R (2013). The regulation of food intake by the gut-brain axis: implications for obesity. *Int Journal of Obesity*, 37:625-633.

[92] Coll A P & Yeo G S H (2013). The hypothalamus and metabolism: integrating signals to control energy and glucose homeostasis. Current *Opinion in Pharmacology,* 13: 970-976.

[93] Coll A P & Yeo G S H (2013). The hypothalamus and metabolism: integrating signals to control energy and glucose homeostasis. Current *Opinion in Pharmacology,* 13: 970-976.

[94] Brdakov D, Luckman S M and Verthratsky A (2005). Glucose-sensing neurons of the hypothalamus. *Philos Trans R Soc Lon B: Bio Sci*, 360:2227-2235.

[95] Zhang W, Cline M A & Gilber E R (2014). Hypothalams-adipose tissue crosstalk: neuropeptide Y and the regulation of energy metabolism. *Nutrition & Metabolism*, 11:27.

[96] Kyrou I, Chrousos G, Tsigos C. (2006). Stress, visceral obesity, and metabolic complications. *Ann N Y Acad Sci.*;1083:77-110.

[97] Kyrou I, Chrousos G, Tsigos C. (2006). Stress, visceral obesity, and metabolic complications. *Ann N Y Acad Sc*i. 1083:77-110.

[98] Paredes S & Ribeiro L (2014). Cortisol: the villain in Metabolic Syndrome? Review. *Rev Assoc Med Bras*, 60(1): 84-92.

[99] Warne JP. (2009). Shaping the stress response: Interplay of palatable food choices, glucocorticoids, insulin and abdominal obesity. *Mol Cell Endocrinol*. 300:137-46.

[100] Kyrou I, Tsigos C. (2009). Stress hormones: physiological stress and regulation of metabolism. *Curr Opin Pharmacol*. 9:787-93.

[101] Adam TC, Epel ES. (2007). Stress, eating and the reward system. *Physiol Behav*. 91:449-58.

[102] *Institute of Medicine.*(2005). Dietary reference intakes for energy, carbohydrate, fiber, fat, fatty acids, cholesterol, protein, and amino acids (macronutrients). National Academies Press, Washington, DC.

[103] Eaton SB. 2006. The ancestral human diet: what was it and should it be a paradigm for contemporary nutrition? Proc. Nutr. Soc. **65**:1–6.

[104] Sleeth ML, Thompson EL, Ford HE, Zac-Varghese SE, Frost G. **(**2010). Free fatty acid receptor 2 and nutrient sensing: a proposed role for fibre, fermentable carbohydrates and short-chain fatty acids in appetite regulation. *Nutr. Res. Rev*. **23**:135–145.

[105] Hussain, S. S., and Bloom, S. R. (2013). The regulation of food intake by the gut-brain axis: implications for obesity. *Int. J. Obes. (Lond.)* 37, 625–633.

[106] Lopaschuk G D, Ussher J R and Jaswal J S (2010) Targeting intermediary metabolism in the hypothalamus as a mechanism to regulate appetite. *Pharmacological Reviews*, 62(2): 237-264.

[107] Schwartz M W (2006.) Central Nervous System Regulation of Food Intake. *Obesity,* 14(Supp): 1S-8S.

[108] Habib AM, Richards P, Rogers GJ, Reimann F, Gribble FM. **(**2013). Co-localisation and secretion of glucagon-like peptide 1 and peptide YYfrom primary cultured human L cells. *Diabetologia* **56**:1413–1416.

[109] Savage AP, Adrian TE, Carolan G, Chatterjee VK, Bloom SR. (1987). Effects of peptide YY (Pyy) on mouth to caecum intestinal transit time and on the rate of gastric emptying in healthy volunteers. Gut **28**:166–170.

[110] Frost G S et al (2014). Impacts of plant-based foods in ancestral hominin diets on the metabolism and function of gut microbiota in vitro. *MBio* 5(3): 00853-14.

[111] Frost G S et al (2014). Impacts of plant-based foods in ancestral hominin diets on the metabolism and function of gut microbiota in vitro. *MBio* 5(3): 00853-14.

[112] Krznari´c Z, Vraneši´c Bender D, Kunovi´c A, Kekez D, Stimac D (2012).. Gut microbiota and obesity. *Dig Dis* 30(2):196-200.

[113] Turnbaugh, P. J., Ley, R. E., Mahowald, M. A., Magrini, V., Mardis, E. R., and Gordon, J. I. (2006) An obesity-associated gut microbiome with increased capacity for energy harvest. *Nature* 444, 1027–1031.

[114] Tilg,H.,andKaser,A.(2011).Gutmicrobiome,obesity,andmetabolicdysfunction. *J. Clin.Invest.* 121, 2126–2132.doi:10.1172/JCI58109.

[115] Yadav H, Lee J-H & Lloyd J (2013). Beneficial metabolic effects of a probiotic via butyrate-induced GLP-1 hormone secretion. *J Biol. Chem*, 288:25088-25097.

[116] Yadav H, Lee J-H & Lloyd J (2013). Beneficial metabolic effects of a probiotic via butyrate-induced GLP-1 hormone secretion. *J Biol. Chem*, 288:25088-25097.

[117] Voreades N, Kozil A & Weir T L (2014). Diet and the development of the human intestinal microbiome. *Frontiers in Microbiology*, 5(494): 1-9.

[118] Claesson, M.J.,Jeffery,I.B.,Conde,S.,Power,S.E.,O'Connor,E.M.,Cusack,S., et al.(2012). Gutmicrobiota composition correlates with diet and health in the elderly. *Nature* 488, 178–184.

[119] Voreades N, Kozil A & Weir T L (2014). Diet and the development of the human intestinal microbiome. *Frontiers in Microbiology*, 5(494): 1-9.

[120] Sun Y et al (2013). Stress-induced corticotropin-releasing hormone-mediated NLRP6 inflammasome inhibition and transmissible enteritis in mice. *Gastroenterology*, 1447): 1478-1487.

[121] Hussain, S. S., and Bloom, S. R. (2013). The regulation of food intake by the gut-brain axis: implications for obesity. *Int. J. Obes. (Lond.)* 37, 625–633.

[122] Hussain, S. S., and Bloom, S. R. (2013). The regulation of food intake by the gut-brain axis: implications for obesity. *Int. J. Obes. (Lond.)* 37, 625–633.

[123] Hussain, S. S., and Bloom, S. R. (2013). The regulation of food intake by the gut-brain axis: implications for obesity. *Int. J. Obes. (Lond.)* 37, 625–633.

[124] Kazaks, A., and Stern, J. S. (2003) Obesity: food intake. *Prim. Care* 30: 301–316.

[125] Kyrou I, Chrousos G, Tsigos C. (2006). Stress, visceral obesity, and metabolic complications. *Ann N Y Acad Sci.*;1083:77-110.

[126] Kyrou I, Chrousos G, Tsigos C. (2006). Stress, visceral obesity, and metabolic complications. *Ann N Y Acad Sci.*;1083:77-110.

[127] Kyrou I, Chrousos G, Tsigos C. (2006). Stress, visceral obesity, and metabolic complications. *Ann N Y Acad Sci.*;1083:77-110.

[128] Kyrou I, Tsigos C. (2009). Stress hormones: physiological stress and regulation of metabolism. *Curr Opin Pharmacol.* 9:787-93.

[129] Kyrou I, Chrousos G, Tsigos C. (2006). Stress, visceral obesity, and metabolic complications. *Ann N Y Acad Sci.*;1083:77-110.

[130] Paredes S & Ribeiro L (2014). Cortisol: the villain in Metabolic Syndrome? Review. *Rev Assoc Med Bras*, 60(1): 84-92.

[131] Charmandari E, Tsigos C, Chrousos G. (2005). Endocrinology of the stress response. *Annu Rev Physiol.* 67:259-84.

[132] Walker BR. (2007). Extra-adrenal regeneration of glucocorticoids by 11betahydroxysteroid dehydrogenase type 1: physiological regulator and pharmacological target for energy partitioning. *Proc Nutr Soc.* 66:1-8.

[133] Wamil M, Seckl JR. (2007). Inhibition of 11beta-hydroxysteroid dehydrogenase type 1 as a promising therapeutic target. Drug Discov Today. 12:504-20.

[134] Shively CA, Laber-Laird K, Anton RF. (1997). Behavior and physiology of social stress and depression in female cynomolgus monkeys. Biol Psychiatry. 41:871-82.

[135] Charmandari E, Tsigos C, Chrousos G. (2005). Endocrinology of the stress response. *Annu Rev Physiol.* 67:259-84.

[136] Paredes S & Ribeiro L (2014). Cortisol: the villain in Metabolic Syndrome? Review. *Rev Assoc Med Bras*, 60(1): 84-92.

[137] Anagnostis P, Athyros VG, Tziomalos K, Karagiannis A, Mikhailidis DP. (2009). Clinical review: the pathogenetic role of cortisol in the metabolic syndrome: a hypothesis. J Clin Endocrinol Metab. 94:2692-701

[138] Warne JP. (2009). Shaping the stress response: Interplay of palatable food choices, glucocorticoids, insulin and abdominal obesity. *Mol Cell Endocrinol.* 300:137-46.

[139] Kyrou I, Chrousos G, Tsigos C. (2006). Stress, visceral obesity, and metabolic complications. *Ann N Y Acad Sci.*;1083:77-110.

[140] Adam TC, Epel ES. (2007). Stress, eating and the reward system. *Physiol Behav.* 91:449-58.

[140] Warne JP. (2009). Shaping the stress response: Interplay of palatable food choices, glucocorticoids, insulin and abdominal obesity. *Mol Cell Endocrinol.* 300:137-46.

[141] Charmandari E, Tsigos C, Chrousos G. (2005). Endocrinology of the stress response. *Annu Rev Physiol.* 67:259-84.

[142] Wang M. (2005) The role of glucocorticoid action in the pathophysiology of the Metabolic Syndrome. *Nutr Metab (Lond)*, 2:3.

[143] Wang M. (2005) The role of glucocorticoid action in the pathophysiology of the Metabolic Syndrome. *Nutr Metab (Lond)*, 2:3.

[144] Tsigos C, Chrousos GP. (2002). Hypothalamic–pituitary–adrenal axis, neuroendocrine factors and stress. J Psychosom Res. 53:865-71.

[145] W.-W. Lin and M. Karin, "A cytokine-mediated link between innate immunity, inflammation, and cancer," *Journal of Clinical Investigation*, vol. 117, no. 5, pp. 1175–1183, 2007.

[146] Elenkov I J (2004). Glucocorticoids and the Th1/Th2 balance. *Ann NY Acad Sci,* 1024: 138-46.

[147] Galon J et al (2002). Gene profiling reveals unknown enhancing and suppressive actions of glucocorticoids on immune cells. *The FASEB Journal*, 16(1): 61-71.

[148] Tian R et al (2014). A possible change process of inflammatory cytokines in the prolonged chronic stress and its ultimate implications for health. Review. *The Scientific World Journal*, Art ID 780616.

[149] Shoelson SE, Herrero L, Naaz A: Obesity, inflammation, and insulin resistance. Gastroenterol 2007, 132:2169–2180.

[150] W.-W. Lin and M. Karin, "A cytokine-mediated link between innate immunity, inflammation, and cancer," *Journal of Clinical Investigation*, vol. 117, no. 5, pp. 1175–1183, 2007.

[151] Tian R et al (2014). A possible change process of inflammatory cytokines in the prolonged chronic stress and its ultimate implications for health. Review. *The Scientific World Journal*, Art ID 780616.

[152] N. Rohleder, "Stimulation of systemic low-grade inflammation by psychosocial stress," *Psychosomatic Medicine*, vol. 76, no. 3, pp. 181–189, 2014.

[153] Tian R et al (2014). A possible change process of inflammatory cytokines in the prolonged chronic stress and its ultimate implications for health. Review. *The Scientific World Journal*, Art ID 780616.

[154] Straub R H (2004). Interaction of the endocrine system with inflammation: a function of energy and volume regulation. Review. *Arthritis Research & Therapy*, 16: 203.

[155] Straub R H (2004). Interaction of the endocrine system with inflammation: a function of energy and volume regulation. Review. *Arthritis Research & Therapy*, 16: 203.

[156] Moller DE, Kaufman KD. Metabolic syndrome: a clinical and molecular perspective. Annu Rev Med. 2005; 56:45-62.

[157] Kelly GS Peripheral metabolism of thyroid hormones. A review. Altern Med Rev 2000, 5 (4):306-33 2.

[158] Kelly G S (2000). Peripheral metabolism of thyroid hormones: A review. *Alternative Medicine Review*, 5(4): 306-333.

[159] Kelly G S (2000). Peripheral metabolism of thyroid hormones: A review. *Alternative Medicine Review*, 5(4): 306-333.

[160] Kelly G S (2000). Peripheral metabolism of thyroid hormones: A review. *Alternative Medicine Review*, 5(4): 306-333.

[161] Kelly G S (2000). Peripheral metabolism of thyroid hormones: A review. *Alternative Medicine Review*, 5(4): 306-333.

[162] Kelly G S (2000). Peripheral metabolism of thyroid hormones: A review. *Alternative Medicine Review*, 5(4): 306-333.

[163] Kelly G S (2000). Peripheral metabolism of thyroid hormones: A review. *Alternative Medicine Review*, 5(4): 306-333.

[164] Iwen A et al (2013). Thyroid hormones and the metabolic syndrome. *Eur Thyroid J,* 2: 83-92.

[165] Ohnhaus EE, Studer H. A link between liver microsomal enzyme activity and thyroid hormone metabolism in man. *Br J Clin Pharmacol* 1983;15:71-76.

[166] Garcia-Ruiz C, Kaplowitz N & Fernadez-Checa J C (2013). Role of mitochondria in alcoholic liver disease. *Curr Pathobiol Rep*, 1(3): 159-168.

[167] Voet, Donald; Judith G. Voet, Charlotte W. Pratt. Fundamentals of Biochemistry, 2nd Edition. 2006. John Wiley and Sons, Inc. p. 547.

[168] Liesa M & Shirihai O S (2013). Mitochondrial dynamics in the regulation of nutrient utilisation and energy expenditure. Review. *Cell Metabolism*, 17: 491-506.

[169] Patti M-E, Corvera S: The role of mitochondria in the pathogenesis of type 2 diabetes. Endocrine Rev 2010, 31:364–395.

[170] Lee H K (2011). Mitochondrial dysfunction and insulin resistance: The contribution of dioxin-like substances. *Diabetes Metab J*, 25: 207-215.

[171] Zhan M et al (2013). Mitochondrial dynamics: regulatory mechanisms and emerging role in renal pathophysiology. *Kidney Int*, 83(4): 568-581.

[172] Liesa M & Shirihai O S (2013). Mitochondrial dynamics in the regulation of nutrient utilisation and energy expenditure. Review. *Cell Metabolism*, 17: 491-506.

[173] Liesa M & Shirihai O S (2013). Mitochondrial dynamics in the regulation of nutrient utilisation and energy expenditure. Review. *Cell Metabolism*, 17: 491-506.

[174] Liesa M & Shirihai O S (2013). Mitochondrial dynamics in the regulation of nutrient utilisation and energy expenditure. Review. *Cell Metabolism*, 17: 491-506.

[175] Gomes, L.C., Di Benedetto, G., and Scorrano, L. (2011). During autophagy mitochondria elongate, are spared from degradation and sustain cell viability. Nat. Cell Biol. 13, 589–598.

[176] Liesa M & Shirihai O S (2013). Mitochondrial dynamics in the regulation of nutrient utilisation and energy expenditure. Review. *Cell Metabolism*, 17: 491-506.

[177] Zhan M et al (2013). Mitochondrial dynamics: regulatory mechanisms and emerging role in renal pathophysiology. *Kidney Int*, 83(4): 568-581.

[178] Alam A & Rahman M (2014). Mitochondrial dysfunction in obesity: potential benefit and mechanism of co-enzyme Q10 supplementation in metabolic syndrome. *Journal of Diabetes & Metabolic Disorders*, 13:60.

[179] Lelli JL, Becks LL, Dabrowska MI, Hinshaw DB (1998). "ATP converts necrosis to apoptosis in oxidant-injured endothelial cells". *Free Radic. Biol. Med.* **25** (6): 694–702.

[180] Lee H K (2011). Mitochondrial dysfunction and insulin resistance: The contribution of dioxin-like substances. *Diabetes Metab J*, 25: 207-215.

[181] http://chm.pops.int/convention/tabid/54/language/en-US/Default.aspx.

[182] Lee DH, Lee IK, Porta M, Steffes M, Jacobs DR Jr. Relationship between serum concentrations of persistent organic pollutants and the prevalence of metabolic syndrome among non-diabetic adults: results from the National Health and Nutrition Examination Survey 1999-2002. Diabetologia 2007;50:1841-51.

[183] US Deptartment of Health and Human services, Agency for Toxic substance and Disease Registry (ATSDR), CERCLApriority list of substances, 2007.

[184] Sharma B, Singh S & Siddiqi N J (2014). Biomedical implications of heavy metals induced imbalances in redox systems. Review. *BioMed Research International*, Article ID 640754.

[185] Sharma B, Singh S & Siddiqi N J (2014). Biomedical implications of heavy metals induced imbalances in redox systems. Review. *BioMed Research International*, Article ID 640754.

[186] Myhill S (2014). It's mitochondria not hypochondria: detox in the treatment of chronic fatigue. *CAM* Oct: 12-14.

[187] Sharma B, Singh S & Siddiqi N J (2014). Biomedical implications of heavy metals induced imbalances in redox systems. Review. *BioMed Research International*, Article ID 640754.

[188] Sharma B, Singh S & Siddiqi N J (2014). Biomedical implications of heavy metals induced imbalances in redox systems. Review. *BioMed Research International*, Article ID 640754.

[189] Sharma B, Singh S & Siddiqi N J (2014). Biomedical implications of heavy metals induced imbalances in redox systems. Review. *BioMed Research International*, Article ID 640754.

[190] Myhill S (2014). It's mitochondria not hypochondria: detox in the treatment of chronic fatigue. *CAM* Oct: 12-14.

[191] Sharma B, Singh S & Siddiqi N J (2014). Biomedical implications of heavy metals induced imbalances in redox systems. Review. *BioMed Research International*, Article ID 640754.

[192] Kleiner S M (1999) Water: an essential but overlooked nutrient. J Am Dietetic Assoc, 99(2): 200-206.

[193] Kleiner S M (1999) Water: an essential but overlooked nutrient. J Am Dietetic Assoc, 99(2): 200-206.

[194] Zhang Y et al (2014). Cafeeine and diuresis during rest and exercise: A meta-analysis. *J Sci Med Sport,* S1440-2440(14): 00143-1.

[195] Hew-Butler T et al (2008). Osmotic and nonosmotic regulation of arginine vasopressin during prolonged endurance exercise. **J Clin Endocrinol Metab**, 93(6): 2072-2078.

[196] Centres for Disease Control and Prevention. Insufficient sleep in a public health epidemic. http://www.cdc.gov/features/dssleep/index.html#References. [Accessed 22/11/14].

[197] NHS Choices. Why lack of sleep is bad for your health. http://www.nhs.uk/livewell/tiredness-and-fatigue/pages/lack-of-sleep-health-risks.aspx. [Accessed 22/11/14].

[198] Cirelli C, Tononi G. Is sleep essential? PLoS Biol. 2008;6(8): e216.

[199] Belenky G, Wesensten NJ, Thorne DR, et al. Patterns of performance degradation and restoration during sleep restriction and

subsequent recovery: a sleep dose–response study. J Sleep Res. 2003;12(1):1–12.

[200] Spiegel K, Leproult R, Van Cauter E. Impact of sleep debt on metabolic and endocrine function. Lancet. 1999;354(9188): 1435–9.

[201] Spiegel K, Tasali E, Penev P, et al. Brief communication: sleep curtailment in healthy young men is associated with decreased leptin levels, elevated ghrelin levels, and increased hunger and appetite. Ann Intern Med. 2004;141(11):846–50.

[202] Krueger JM, Majde JA, Rector DM. Cytokines in immune function and sleep regulation. Handbook Clin Neurol. 2011;98: 229–40.

[203] **Institute of Medicine. *Sleep Disorders and Sleep Deprivation: An Unmet Public Health Problem*. Washington, DC: The National Academies Press; 2006.**

[204] Van Dongen HP, Maislin G, Mullington JM, et al. The cumulative cost of additional wakefulness: dose–response effects on neurobehavioral functions and sleep physiology from chronic sleep restriction and total sleep deprivation. Sleep. 2003;26(2): 117–26.

[205] Tsang A, Barclay J L & Oster H (2014). Interactions between endocrine and circadian systems. Review. *Journal of Molecular Endocrinology*, 52:R1-R16.

[206] Tsang A, Barclay J L & Oster H (2014). Interactions between endocrine and circadian systems. Review. *Journal of Molecular Endocrinology*, 52:R1-R16.

[207] Rea M S (2012). Relationship of morning cortisol to circadian phase and rising time in young adults with delayed sleep time. *International Journal of Endocrinology*, Art AD 749460.

[208] Rea M S (2012). Relationship of morning cortisol to circadian phase and rising time in young adults with delayed sleep time. *International Journal of Endocrinology*, Art AD 749460.

[209] Tsang A, Barclay J L & Oster H (2014). Interactions between endocrine and circadian systems. Review. *Journal of Molecular Endocrinology*, 52:R1-R16.

[210] Kyrou I, Chrousos G, Tsigos C. Stress, visceral obesity, and metabolic complications. Ann N Y Acad Sci. 2006;1083:77-110.

[211] Zisapel N, Tarrasch R & Laudon M (2005). The relationship between melatonin and cortisol rhythms: clinical implications of melatonin therapy. *Drug Development Research*, 65(3): 119-125.

[212] Tsang A, Barclay J L & Oster H (2014). Interactions between endocrine and circadian systems. Review. *Journal of Molecular Endocrinology*, 52:R1-R16.

[213] Figueiro MG, Rea MS, Bullough JD (2006). "Does architectural lighting contribute to breast cancer?". *J Carcinog* **5**: 20

[214] Tsang A, Barclay J L & Oster H (2014). Interactions between endocrine and circadian systems. Review. *Journal of Molecular Endocrinology*, 52:R1-R16.

[215] Waterhouse J, Nevill A, Finnegan J, Williams P, Edwards B, Kao SY & Reilly T 2005 Further assessments of the relationship between jet lag and some of its symptoms. Chronobiology International 22 121–136.

[216] Baron KG, Reid KJ, Kern AS & Zee PC 2011 Role of sleep timing in caloric intake and BMI. Obesity 19 1374–1381.

[217] Doane LD, Kremen WS, Eaves LJ, Eisen SA, Hauger R, Hellhammer D, Levine S, Lupien S, Lyons MJ, Mendoza S et al. 2010 Associations between jet lag and cortisol diurnal rhythms after domestic travel. Health Psychology 29 117–123.

[218] Dijk DJ, Duffy JF, Silva EJ, Shanahan TL, Boivin DB & Czeisler CA 2012 Amplitude reduction and phase shifts of melatonin, cortisol and other circadian rhythms after a gradual advance of sleep and light exposure in humans. PLoS ONE 7 e30037

[219] Kim M J, Lee J H & Duffy J F (2013). Circadian rhythm disorders. *J Clin Outcomes Manag*, 20(11): 513-528.

[220] Kim M J, Lee J H & Duffy J F (2013). Circadian rhythm disorders. *J Clin Outcomes Manag*, 20(11): 513-528.

[221] Bhanu P K & Auger R R (2011). Jetlag and shift-work disorders: how to reset the internal clock. *Cleveland Clinic Journal of Medicine*, 78(10): 675-684.

[222] Gander PH, Gregory KB, Miller DL, Graeber RC, Connell LJ, Rosekind MR. Flight crew fatigue V: Long-haul air transport operations. Aviat Space Environ Med. 1998; 69:B37–B48. [

[223] Pukkala E, Helminen M, Haldorsen T, et al. Cancer incidence among Nordic airline cabin crew. Int J Cancer. 2012; 131:2886–97.

[224] United States Department of Labor Bureau of Labor Statistics. The employment situation - August 2012. Washington, D.C.: U.S. Department of Labor; 2012.

[225] HSE (2011). Changes in shift work patterns over the last 10 years (199-2009). *HSE Research Report* RR887.

[226] Institute of Medicine. *Sleep Disorders and Sleep Deprivation: An Unmet Public Health Problem*. Washington, DC: The National Academies Press; 2006.

[227] Harvard Health (2015). How to sleep better: Tips for getting a good night's sleep. www.helpguide.org. [Accessed 07/01/15].

[228] Harvard Health (2015). Stress Management: How to reduce, prevent and cope with stress. www.helpguide.org. [Accessed 07/01/15].

[229] Puddu A et al (2014). Evidence for the Gut Microbiota Short-Chain Fatty Acids as Key Pathophysiological Molecules Improving Diabetes. *Mediators of Inflammation*, Art ID 162021.

[230] Puddu A et al (2014). Evidence for the Gut Microbiota Short-Chain Fatty Acids as Key Pathophysiological Molecules Improving Diabetes. *Mediators of Inflammation*, Art ID 162021.

[231] M. A. C. Looijer-van Langen and L. A. Dieleman, "Prebiotics in chronic intestinal inflammation," *Inflammatory Bowel Diseases*, vol. 15, no. 3, pp. 454–462, 2009.

[232] Puddu A et al (2014). Evidence for the Gut Microbiota Short-Chain Fatty Acids as Key Pathophysiological Molecules Improving Diabetes. *Mediators of Inflammation*, Art ID 162021.

[233] Puddu A et al (2014). Evidence for the Gut Microbiota Short-Chain Fatty Acids as Key Pathophysiological Molecules Improving Diabetes. *Mediators of Inflammation*, Art ID 162021.

[234] Simopoulous A P (2013). Dietary Omega-3 Fatty Acid Deficiency and High Fructose Intake in the Development of Metabolic Syndrome, Brain Metabolic Abnormalities, and Non-Alcoholic Fatty Liver Disease. *Nutrients*, 5:2901-2923.

[235] Pesta D H & Samuel V T (2014). A high-protein diet for reducing body fat: mechanisms and possible caveats. *Nutrition & Metabolism*, 11:53.

[236] Moran TH, Kinzig KP: Gastrointestinal satiety signals II. Cholecystokinin. Am J Physiol Gastrointest Liver Physiol 2004, 286:G183–G188.

[237] Veldhorst M, Smeets A, Soenen S, Hochstenbach-Waelen A, Hursel R, Diepvens K, Lejeune M, Luscombe-Marsh N, Westerterp-Plantenga M: Protein-induced satiety: effects and mechanisms of different proteins. Physiol Behav 2008, 94:300–307.

[238] Pesta D H & Samuel V T (2014). A high-protein diet for reducing body fat: mechanisms and possible caveats. *Nutrition & Metabolism*, 11:53.

[239] Petzke K J et al (2014). Beyond the Role of Dietary Protein and Amino Acids in the Prevention of Diet-Induced Obesity. Int J Mol Sci, 15: 1374-1391.

[240] Simopoulous A P (2013). Dietary Omega-3 Fatty Acid Deficiency and High Fructose Intake in the Development of Metabolic Syndrome, Brain Metabolic Abnormalities, and Non-Alcoholic Fatty Liver Disease. *Nutrients*, 5:2901-2923.

[241] Simopoulous A P (2013). Dietary Omega-3 Fatty Acid Deficiency and High Fructose Intake in the Development of Metabolic Syndrome, Brain Metabolic Abnormalities, and Non-Alcoholic Fatty Liver Disease. *Nutrients*, 5:2901-2923.

[242] Tsang A H et al (2014). Interactions between endocrine and circadian systems. *Journal of Molecular Endocrinology*, 52: R1-R16.

[243] Hirao J, Arakawa S, Watanabe K, Ito K & Furukawa T 2006 Effects of restricted feeding on daily fluctuations of hepatic functions including p450 monooxygenase activities in rats. Journal of Biological Chemistry 281 3165–3171

[244] Hirao J, Arakawa S, Watanabe K, Ito K & Furukawa T 2006 Effects of restricted feeding on daily fluctuations of hepatic functions including p450 monooxygenase activities in rats. Journal of Biological Chemistry 281 3165–3171

[245] Tsang A H et al (2014). Interactions between endocrine and circadian systems. *Journal of Molecular Endocrinology*, 52: R1-R16.

[246] LeSauter J, Hoque N, Weintraub M, Pfaff DW & Silver R 2009 Stomach ghrelin-secreting cells as food-entrainable circadian clocks. PNAS 106 13582–13587.

[247] Lawrence F (2005). *Not on the label: What really goes into the food on your plate*. USA, California: Penguin Group.

[248] www.canada.com. Top 10 most common environmental toxins. [Accessed 02/02/15].

[249] Fairfield K M & Fletcher R H (2002). Vitamins for chronic disease prevention in adults: Scientific Review. *JAMA*, 287(23): 3116-3126.

[250] Willett W C & Stamfer M J (2001). Clinical Practice: What vitamins should I be taking, doctor? *N Engl J Med*, 245(25): 1819-24.

[251] Bronstein A C et al (2011). 2010 Annual report of the American Association of Poison Control Centre's National Poison Data System (NPDS): 28th Ann Report. *Clin Toxicol*, 49(10): 910-941.

[252] CDC (2015). Prescription drug overdose in the US: Fact Sheet. www.cdc.gov/homeandrecreationalsafety/overdose/facts.html. [Accessed 02/02/15].

[253] CDC (2015). Prescription drug overdose in the US: Fact Sheet. www.cdc.gov/homeandrecreationalsafety/overdose/facts.html. [Accessed 02/02/15].

[254] Niedzwiecki A. Commentary on the Safety of Vitamins. [Accessed 02/02/15]. http://www4.dr-rath-foundation.org/NHC/articles/2013_08_16_commentary_safety_vitamins.html

[255] NHS Choices (2011). Supplements, who needs them? http://www.nhs.uk/news/2011/05May/Documents/BtH_supplements.pdf. [Accessed 02/02/15].

[256] (2015) *Nutritional Supplements in the US, 6th Ed*. US, Market Research Group LLC: Packaged Facts.

[257] Traber M G et al (1998). Synthetic as compared with natural vitamin E is preferentially excreted as alpha CEHC in human urine: studies using deuterated alpha-tocopheryl acetates. *FEBS Lett*, 437(1-2): 145-8.

[258] Ward E (2014). Addressing nutritional gaps with multivitamin and mineral supplements. *Nutr J*. 13:72.

[259] Prentice RL. Clinical trials and observational studies to assess the chronic disease benefits and risks of multivitamin-multimineral supplements. Am J Clin Nutr. 2007;85:308S–313S

[260] Bailey RL, Fulgoni VL III, Keast DR, Dwyer JT. Examination of vitamin intakes among US adults by dietary supplement use. J Acad Nutr Diet. 2012;112:657–663.

[261] Troesch B, Hoeft B, McBurney M, Eggersdorfer M, Weber P. Dietary surveys indicate vitamin intakes below recommendations are common in representative Western countries. Br J Nutr.2012;108:692–698

[262] Krznarić Z, Vranešić Bender D, Kunović A, Kekez D, Stimac D (2012).. Gut microbiota and obesity. *Dig Dis* 30(2):196-200.

[263] Festi D et al (2014). Gut microbiota & metabolic syndrome. *World J Gastroenterol*, 20(43): 16079-16094.

[264] Festi D et al (2014). Gut microbiota & metabolic syndrome. *World J Gastroenterol*, 20(43): 16079-16094.

[265] Festi D et al (2014). Gut microbiota & metabolic syndrome. *World J Gastroenterol*, 20(43): 16079-16094.

[266] Festi D et al (2014). Gut microbiota & metabolic syndrome. *World J Gastroenterol*, 20(43): 16079-16094.

[267] Wall R et al (2009). Metabolic activity of the enteric microbiota influences the fatty acid composition of murine and porcine liver and adipose tissues. *Am J Clin Nutr*; **89**: 1393-1401.

[268] Festi D et al (2014). Gut microbiota & metabolic syndrome. *World J Gastroenterol*, 20(43): 16079-16094.

[269] Festi D et al (2014). Gut microbiota & metabolic syndrome. *World J Gastroenterol*, 20(43): 16079-16094.

[270] Iacono A, Raso GM, Canani RB, Calignano A, Meli R. Probiotics as an emerging therapeutic strategy to treat NAFLD: focus on molecular and biochemical mechanisms. *J Nutr Biochem* 2011; **22**: 699-711

[271] Khani, S.; Hosseini, H.M.; Taheri, M.; Nourani, M.R.; Imani Fooladi, A.A. Probiotics as an alternative strategy for prevention and treatment of human diseases: A review. Inflamm. Allergy Drug Targets 2012, 11, 79–89.

[272] Festi D et al (2014). Gut microbiota & metabolic syndrome. *World J Gastroenterol*, 20(43): 16079-16094.

[273] El-Lakkany N M (2012). Anti-inflammatory/anti-fibrotic effects of the hepatoprotective silymarin and the schistosomicide praziquantel against schistosoma mansoni-induced liver fibrosis. *Parasites & Vectors*, 5:9.

[274] Duarte S et al (2015). Matrix metalloproteinases in liver injury, repair and fibrosis. *Matrix Biology*, doi: 10.1016/j.matbio.2015.01.004

[275] Ramadori G et al (2008). Physiology and pathology of liver inflammation, damage and repair. *Journal of Physiology and Pharmacology*, 59(1): 107-117.

[276] Duarte S et al (2015). Matrix metalloproteinases in liver injury, repair and fibrosis. *Matrix Biology*, doi: 10.1016/j.matbio.2015.01.004

[277] Sheedfar F et al (2013). Liver diseases and aging: friends or foes? *Aging Cell*, 12:950-954.

[278] Sheedfar F et al (2013). Liver diseases and aging: friends or foes? *Aging Cell*, 12:950-954.

[279] Sheedfar F et al (2013). Liver diseases and aging: friends or foes? *Aging Cell*, 12:950-954.

[280] Sheedfar F et al (2013). Liver diseases and aging: friends or foes? *Aging Cell*, 12:950-954.

[281] Xiao J et al (2013). Recent advances in the herbal treatment of non-alcoholic fatty liver disease. *J Tradit Complement Med*, 3(2): 88-94.

[282] Sheedfar F et al (2013). Liver diseases and aging: friends or foes? *Aging Cell*, 12:950-954.

[283] Xiao J et al (2013). Recent advances in the herbal treatment of non-alcoholic fatty liver disease. *J Tradit Complement Med*, 3(2): 88-94.

[284] El-Lakkany N M (2012). Anti-inflammatory/anti-fibrotic effects of the hepatoprotective silymarin and the schistosomicide praziquantel against schistosoma mansoni-induced liver fibrosis. *Parasites & Vectors*, 5:9.

[285] Xiao J et al (2013). Recent advances in the herbal treatment of non-alcoholic fatty liver disease. *J Tradit Complement Med*, 3(2): 88-94.

[286] Pais P & D'Amato M (2014). In vivo efficacy study of milk thistle extract (ETHIS-094) in STAM model of non-alcoholic steatohepatitis. *Drugs R D*, 14:291-299.

[287] Milosevic N et al (2014). Phytotherapy and NAFLD – from goals and challenges to clinical practice. *Rev Recent Clin Trials*, 9(3): 195-203.

[288] Milosevic N et al (2014). Phytotherapy and NAFLD – from goals and challenges to clinical practice. *Rev Recent Clin Trials*, 9(3): 195-203.

[289] Aguirre R & May J M (2008). Inflammation in the vascular bed: Importance of vitamin C. *Pharmacol Ther*, 119(1): 96-103.

[290] Ipsen D H et al (2014). Does vitamin C deficiency promote fatty liver disease development? *Nutrients*, 6: 5473-5499.

[291] Ipsen D H et al (2014). Does vitamin C deficiency promote fatty liver disease development? *Nutrients*, 6: 5473-5499.

[292] Lykkesfeldt, J.; Poulsen, H.E. (2010). Is vitamin C supplementation beneficial? Lessons learned from randomised controlled trials. *Br. J. Nutr. 103*, 1251–1259.

[293] Johnston, C.S.; Beezhold, B.L.; Mostow, B.; Swan, P.D. Plasma vitamin C is inversely related to body mass index and waist circumference but not to plasma adiponectin in nonsmoking adults. *J. Nutr.* **2007**, *137*, 1757–1762.

[294] Ipsen D H et al (2014). Does vitamin C deficiency promote fatty liver disease development? *Nutrients*, 6: 5473-5499.

[295] W.-W. Lin and M. Karin, "A cytokine-mediated link between innate immunity, inflammation, and cancer," *Journal of Clinical Investigation*, vol. 117, no. 5, pp. 1175–1183, 2007.

[296] Deruelle F & Baron B (2008). Vitamin C: Is supplementation necessary for optimal health? *J Altern Complement Med*, 14(10): 1291-8.

[297] Aguirre R & May J M (2008). Inflammation in the vascular bed: Importance of vitamin C. *Pharmacol Ther*, 119(1): 96-103.

[298] Paoletti R et al (2006). Metabolic syndrome, inflammation and atherosclerosis. *Vasc Health Risk Manag*, 2(2): 1450152.

[299] NHS (2015). Atherosclerosis. http://www.nhs.uk/Conditions/Atherosclerosis/Pages/Introduction.aspx. [Accessed 04/02/15].

[300] American Heart Association (2015). Heart disease and stroke statistics – At a Glance. http://www.heart.org/idc/groups/ahamah-public/@wcm/@sop/@smd/documents/downloadable/ucm_470704.pdf. [Accessed 04/02/15].

[301] Aguirre R & May J M (2008). Inflammation in the vascular bed: Importance of vitamin C. *Pharmacol Ther*, 119(1): 96-103.

[302] Aguirre R & May J M (2008). Inflammation in the vascular bed: Importance of vitamin C. *Pharmacol Ther*, 119(1): 96-103.

[303] Deruelle F & Baron B (2008). Vitamin C: Is supplementation necessary for optimal health? *J Altern Complement Med*, 14(10): 1291-8.

[304] Afkhami-Ardekani, M.; Shojaoddiny-Ardekani, A. Effect of vitamin C on blood glucose, serum lipids & serum insulin in type 2 diabetes patients. *Indian J. Med. Res.* 2007, *126*, 471–474.

[305] Barbagallo, M.; Dominguez, L.J.; Galioto, A.; Ferlisi, A.; Cani, C.; Malfa, L.; Pineo, A.; Busardo, A.; Paolisso, G. Role of magnesium in insulin action, diabetes and cardio-metabolic syndrome X. *Mol. Asp. Med.* 2003, *24*, 39–52.

[306] Igamberdiev A U & Kleczkowski L A (2015). Optimisation of APT synthase function in mitochondria and chloroplasts via the adenylate kinase equilibrium. *Frontiers in Plant Science*, 6(10): 1-8.

[307] Takaya J, Higashino H, Kobayashi Y. Intracellular magnesium and insulin resistance. Magnes Res. 2004;17:126–36.

[308] Chubanov V, Gudermann T, Schlingmann KP. Essential role for TRPM6 in epithelial magnesium transport and body magnesium homeostasis. Pflugers Arch. 2005;451:228–34.

[309] Volpe S L (2013). Magnesium in Disease Prevention and Overall Health. *American Society for Nutrition*. *Adv Nutr*, 4:378S-383S.

[310] Nielsen FH: Magnesium, inflammation, and obesity in chronic disease. Nutr Rev 2010, 68(6):333–340.

[311] Ju S-Y et al (2014). Dietary magnesium intake and metabolic syndrome in the adult population: Dose-response meta-analysis and meta-regression. *Nutrients*, 6: 6005-6019.

[312] Volpe S L (2013). Magnesium in Disease Prevention and Overall Health. *American Society for Nutrition*. *Adv Nutr*, 4:378S-383S.

[313] Stebbing JB et al. Reactive hypoglycemia and magnesium. Magnesium Bull 1982; 2:131–4.

[314] Held K et al. Oral Mg supplementation reverse age-related neuroendocrine and sleep EEG changes in humans. Pharmacopsychiatry 2002; 35(4):135-43.

[315] Hadjistavri, L.S.; Sarafidis, P.A.; Georgianos, P.I.; Tziolas, I.M.; Aroditis, C.P.; Hitoglou-Makedou, A.; Zebekakis, P.E.; Pikilidou, M.I.; Lasaridis, A.N. Beneficial effects of oral magnesium supplementation on insulin sensitivity and serum lipid profile. *Med. Sci. Monit.* **2010**, *16*, CR307–CR312.

[316] Setaro L et al (2014). Magnesium status and the physical performance of volleyball players: effects of magnesium supplementation. *J Sports Sci*, 32(5): 438-45.

[317] NIH (2015). Calcium: Dietary supplement factsheet. http://ods.od.nih,gov.factsheets. [Accessed 15/02/15].

[318] Cardenas C et al (2010). Essential regulation of cell bioenergetics by constitutive InsP$_3$. *Cell*, 142(2): 270-283.

[319] Cardenas C et al (2010). Essential regulation of cell bioenergetics by constitutive InsP$_3$. *Cell*, 142(2): 270-283.

[320] Igamberdiev A U & Kleczkowski L A (2015). Optimisation of APT synthase function in mitochondria and chloroplasts via the adenylate kinase equilibrium. *Frontiers in Plant Science*, 6(10): 1-8.

[321] Torres M R S G & Sanjuliani A F (2012). Does calcium intake affect cardiovascular risk factor and/or events? *CLINICS*, 67(7): 839-844.

[322] Huang J-H et al (2014). High or low calcium intake increases cardiovascular disease risks in older patients with type 2 diabetes. *Cardiovascular Diabetology*, 13: 120.

[323] Huang J-H et al (2014). High or low calcium intake increases cardiovascular disease risks in older patients with type 2 diabetes. *Cardiovascular Diabetology*, 13: 120.

[324] Depeint F et al (2006). Mitochondrial function and toxicity: role of B vitamins on mitochondrial energy metabolism. *Chemico-Biological Interactions*, 163(1-2): 94-112.

[325] Stough C, Scholey A, Lloyd J, Spong J, Myers S, Downey LA. The effect of 90 day administration of a high dose vitamin B-complex on work stress. Human Psychopharmacol. 2011;26:470–476

[326] Chamorro-Premuzic T, Ahmetoglu G, Furnham A. Little more than personality: Dispositional determinants of test anxiety (the Big Five, core self-evaluations, and self-assessed intelligence) Learn Individ Differ. 2008;18:258–263

[327] Angelo G (2013). What is metabolism? http://lpi.oregonstate.edu/ss13/metabolism.html Linus Pauling Institute. [Accessed 15/02/15].

[328] Depeint F et al (2006). Mitochondrial function and toxicity: role of B vitamins on mitochondrial energy metabolism. *Chemico-Biological Interactions*, 163(1-2): 94-112.

[329] Golbidi S et al (2011). Diabetes and alpha-lipoic acid. *Frontiers in Pharmacology*, 2(69): 1-15.

[330] Golbidi S et al (2011). Diabetes and alpha-lipoic acid. *Frontiers in Pharmacology*, 2(69): 1-15.

[331] Chen L & Yang G (2014). PPARs integrate the mammalian clock and energy metabolism. Review. *PPAR Research*, ID 653017.

[332] Golbidi S et al (2011). Diabetes and alpha-lipoic acid. *Frontiers in Pharmacology*, 2(69): 1-15.

[333] Golbidi S et al (2011). Diabetes and alpha-lipoic acid. *Frontiers in Pharmacology*, 2(69): 1-15.

[334] Kola,B.,Boscaro,M.,Rutter,G.A., Grossman,A.B.,andKorbonits,M. (2006). ExpandingroleofAMPK in endocrinology. TrendsEndocrinol. Metab. 17, 205–215.

[335] Golbidi S et al (2011). Diabetes and alpha-lipoic acid. *Frontiers in Pharmacology*, 2(69): 1-15.

[336] Chen L & Yang G (2014). PPARs integrate the mammalian clock and energy metabolism. Review. *PPAR Research*, ID 653017.

[337] Golbidi S et al (2011). Diabetes and alpha-lipoic acid. *Frontiers in Pharmacology*, 2(69): 1-15.

[338] Chen L & Yang G (2014). PPARs integrate the mammalian clock and energy metabolism. Review. *PPAR Research*, ID 653017.

[339] Golbidi S et al (2011). Diabetes and alpha-lipoic acid. *Frontiers in Pharmacology*, 2(69): 1-15.

[340] Lee, W.J., Song, K.H. ,Koh, E.H., Won, J.C. ,Kim ,H.S. ,Park ,H.S., Kim, M.S., Kim, S.W. ,Lee, K.U., and Park ,J.Y .(2005a). Alpha-lipoic acid increases insulin sensitivity by activating AMPK in skeletal muscle. *Biochem. Biophys. Res. Commun.* 332, 885–891.

[341] Lee, W.J. ,Koh, E.H., Won, J.C., Kim ,M.S. ,Park J.Y. ,and Lee, K. U.(2005b). .Obesity: the role of hypothalamic AMP-activated protein kinase in body weight regulation. *Int .J .Biochem .Cell Biol.* 37, 2254–2259.

[342] Koh, E.H., Lee, W.J., Lee, S.A., Kim ,E. H., Cho, E.H., Jeong, E., Kim, D.W., Kim, M.S., Park, J.Y., Park, K.G., Lee, H.J., Lee, I.K., Lim, S., Jang, H. C., Lee, K.H., and Lee, K.U. (2011). Effects of alpha-lipoic acid on body weight in obese subjects. *.Am.J.Med.* 124, 851–858.

[343] Ziegler D. Thioctic acid for patients with symptomatic diabetic polyneuropathy: a critical review. Treat Endocrinol. 2004;3(3):173-189.

[344] Flanagan J L, Simmons P A, Vehige J, Wilcox M D P and Garrett Q (2010) Role of carnitine in disease. *Nutrition & Metabolism*, 7:30.

[345] Cha Y-S (2008) Effects of L-carnitine on obesity, diabetes and as an ergogenic aid. *Asia Pacific Journal of Clinical Nutrition*, 17(S1): 306-308.

[346] Noland R C, Koves T R, Seiler S E, Lum H, Lust R M, Ilkayeva O, Stevens R D, Hegardt F G and Muoio D M (2009) Carnitine insufficiency caused by aging and overnutrition compromises mitochondrial performance and metabolic control. *Journal of Biological Chemistry,* 284(34): 22840-22852.

[347] Arrigoni-Martelli E & Caso V. Carnitine protects mitochondria and removes toxic acyls from xenobiotics. .Drugs Exp Clin Res. 2001; 27(1):27-49.

[348] Karlic H and Lohninger A (2004) Supplementation of L-carnitine in athletes: does it make sense? *Nutrition*, 20: 709-715.

[349] Cha Y-S (2008) Effects of L-carnitine on obesity, diabetes and as an ergogenic aid. *Asia Pacific Journal of Clinical Nutrition*, 17(S1): 306-308.

[350] Noland R C, Koves T R, Seiler S E, Lum H, Lust R M, Ilkayeva O, Stevens R D, Hegardt F G and Muoio D M (2009) Carnitine insufficiency caused by aging and overnutrition compromises mitochondrial performance and metabolic control. *Journal of Biological Chemistry*, 284(34): 22840-22852.

[351] Noland R C, Koves T R, Seiler S E, Lum H, Lust R M, Ilkayeva O, Stevens R D, Hegardt F G and Muoio D M (2009) Carnitine insufficiency caused by aging and overnutrition compromises mitochondrial performance and metabolic control. *Journal of Biological Chemistry*, 284(34): 22840-22852.

[352] Flanagan J L, Simmons P A, Vehige J, Wilcox M D P and Garrett Q (2010) Role of carnitine in disease. *Nutrition & Metabolism*, 7:30.

[353] Wolfgang M J, Cha S H, Millington D S, Cline G, Shulman G, Suwa A, Asaumi M, Kurama T, Shimokawa T, and Lane M D (2008) Brain-specific carnitine palmitoyl-transferase-1c: role in CNS fatty acid metabolism, food intake and body weight. *Journal of Neurochemistry*, 105: 1550-1559.

[354] Lopaschuk G D, Ussher J R and Jaswal J S (2010) Targeting intermediary metabolism in the hypothalamus as a mechanism to regulate appetite. *Pharmacological Reviews*, 62(2): 237-264.

[355] Wolfgang M J and Lane M D (2006) The role of hypothalamic malonyl-CoA in energy homeostasis: mini-review. *Journal of Biological Chemistry*, 281(49): 37265-37269.

[356] Lane M D, Wolfgang M, Cha S-H and Dai Y (2008) Regulation of food intake and energy expenditure by hypothalamic malonyl-CoA. *International Journal of Obesity*, 32: S49-S54.

[357] Wolfgang M J, Cha S H, Millington D S, Cline G, Shulman G, Suwa A, Asaumi M, Kurama T, Shimokawa T, and Lane M D (2008) Brain-specific carnitine palmitoyl-transferase-1c: role in CNS fatty acid metabolism, food intake and body weight. *Journal of Neurochemistry,* 105: 1550-1559.

[358] Lopaschuk G D, Ussher J R and Jaswal J S (2010) Targeting intermediary metabolism in the hypothalamus as a mechanism to regulate appetite. *Pharmacological Reviews*, 62(2): 237-264.

[359] Dieguez C, Fruhbeck G and Lopez M (2009) Hypothalamic lipids and the regulation of energy homeostasis. *Obesity Facts,* 2(2): 126-135.

[360] Wolfgang M J, Cha S H, Sidhaye A, Chohnan S, Cline G, Shulman G and Lane M D (2007) Regulation of hypothalamic malonyl-CoA by central glucose and leptin. *PNAS*, 104(49): 19285-19290.

[361] Wolfgang M J, Cha S H, Millington D S, Cline G, Shulman G, Suwa A, Asaumi M, Kurama T, Shimokawa T, and Lane M D (2008) Brain-specific carnitine palmitoyl-transferase-1c: role in CNS fatty acid metabolism, food intake and body weight. *Journal of Neurochemistry*, 105: 1550-1559.

[362] Wolfgang M J and Lane M D (2011) Hypothalamic malonyl-CoA and CPT-1c treatment of obesity. *FEBS Journal*, 278:552-558

[363] Flanagan J L, Simmons P A, Vehige J, Wilcox M D P and Garrett Q (2010) Role of carnitine in disease. *Nutrition & Metabolism*, 7:30.

[364] Shang R, Sun Z and Li H (2014). Effective dosing of L-carnitine in the secondary prevention of CVD: a systematic review and meta-analysis. *Cardiovascular Disorders*, 14:88.

[365] Flanagan JL, Simmons PA, Vehige J, Willcox MD, Garrett Q: Review Role of carnitine in disease. 2010.

[366] Evans AM, Fornasini G: Pharmacokinetics of L-carnitine. Clin Pharmacokinet 2003, 42(11):941–967

[367] Koeth RA, Wang Z, Levison BS, Buffa JA, Sheehy BT, Britt EB, Fu X, Wu Y, Li L, Smith JD, DiDonato JA, Chen J, Li H, Wu GD, Lewis JD, Warrier M, Brown JM, Krauss RM, Tang WH, Bushman FD, Lusis AJ, Hazen SL: Intestinal microbiota metabolism of l-carnitine, a nutrient in red meat, promotes atherosclerosis. Nat Med 2013, 19(5):576–585.

[368] Shang R, Sun Z and Li H (2014). Effective dosing of L-carnitine in the secondary prevention of CVD: a systematic review and meta-analysis. *Cardiovascular Disorders*, 14:88.

[369] Angelo G (2013). What is metabolism? http://lpi.oregonstate.edu/ss13/metabolism.html Linus Pauling Institute. [Accessed 15/02/15].

[370] Quinzii C M & Hirano M (2010). Coenzyme Q and mitochondrial disease. *Dev Disabil Res Rev*, 16(2): 183-188.

[371] Quinzii C M & Hirano M (2010). Coenzyme Q and mitochondrial disease. *Dev Disabil Res Rev*, 16(2): 183-188.

[372] Groneberg D A et al (2005). Coenzyme Q10 affects expression of genes involved in cell signalling, metabolism and transport in human CaCo2 cells. *Int J Biochem Cell Biol*, 37(6): 1208-18.

[373] Lee S K et al (2012). Coenzyme Q10 increases the fatty acid oxidation through AMPK-mediated PPAR-alpha induction in 3T3-L1 preadipocytes. *Cell Signal*, 24(12); 2329-36.

[374] Turunen M, Olsson J, Dallner G. Metabolism and function of coenzyme Q. Biochim Biophys Acta. 2004; 1660:171–199.

[375] Sohal R S & Forster M J (2007). Coenzyme Q, oxidative stress and aging. *Mitochondrion*, 7(supply): S103-S111.

[376] Bergamini C et al (2012). A Water Soluble CoQ10 Formulation Improves Intracellular Distribution and Promotes Mitochondrial Respiration in Cultured Cells. *PLoS ONE*, 7(3): e33712.

[377] Bergamini C et al (2012). A Water Soluble CoQ10 Formulation Improves Intracellular Distribution and Promotes Mitochondrial Respiration in Cultured Cells. *PLoS ONE*, 7(3): e33712.

[378] Quinzii C M & Hirano M (2010). Coenzyme Q and mitochondrial disease. *Dev Disabil Res Rev*, 16(2): 183-188.

[379] Quinzii C M & Hirano M (2010). Coenzyme Q and mitochondrial disease. *Dev Disabil Res Rev*, 16(2): 183-188.

[380] *Garrido-Maraver J,* Cordero MD, Oropesa-Avila M, Vega AF, de la Mata M, Pavon AD, Alcocer-Gomez E, Calero CP, Paz MV, Alanis M, de Lavera I, Cotan D, Sanchez-Alcazar JA. Clinical applications of coenzyme Q10. Front Biosci 2014; **19**: 619-633

[381] Wagner A E et al (2012). A Combination of Lipoic Acid Plus Coenzyme Q10 Induces PGC1α, a Master Switch of Energy Metabolism, Improves Stress Response, and Increases Cellular Glutathione Levels in Cultured C2C12 SkeletalMuscle Cells. *Oxidative Medicine and Cellular Longevity*, Art ID 835970.

[382] Golbidi S et al (2011). Diabetes and alpha-lipoic acid. *Frontiers in Pharmacology*, 2(69): 1-15.

[383] Wagner A E et al (2012). A Combination of Lipoic Acid Plus Coenzyme Q10 Induces PGC1α, a Master Switch of Energy Metabolism, Improves Stress Response, and Increases Cellular Glutathione Levels in Cultured C2C12 SkeletalMuscle Cells. *Oxidative Medicine and Cellular Longevity*, Art ID 835970.

[384] Linus Pauling Institute (2015). Coenzyme Q10. http://lpi.oregonstate.edu/infocenter/othernuts/coq10/. [Accessed 18/02/15].

[385] Owen L & Sunram-Lea S I (2011). Metabolic Agents that Enhance ATP can Improve Cognitive Functioning: A Review of the Evidence for Glucose, Oxygen, Pyruvate, Creatine, and L-Carnitine. *Nutrients*, 3:735-755.

[386] Wallimann T et al (2011). The creatine kinase system and pleiotropic effects of creatine. *Amino Acids*, 40: 1271-1296.

[387] Owen L & Sunram-Lea S I (2011). Metabolic Agents that Enhance ATP can Improve Cognitive Functioning: A Review of the Evidence for Glucose, Oxygen, Pyruvate, Creatine, and L-Carnitine. *Nutrients*, 3:735-755.

[388] Wallimann T et al (2011). The creatine kinase system and pleiotropic effects of creatine. *Amino Acids*, 40: 1271-1296.

[389] Guimaraes-Ferreira L (2014). Role of the phosphocreatine system on energetic homeostasis in skeletal and cardiac muscles. *Einstein* 12(1): 126-31.

[390] Guimaraes-Ferreira L (2014). Role of the phosphocreatine system on energetic homeostasis in skeletal and cardiac muscles. *Einstein* 12(1): 126-31.

[391] Guimaraes-Ferreira L (2014). Role of the phosphocreatine system on energetic homeostasis in skeletal and cardiac muscles. *Einstein* 12(1): 126-31.

[392] Guimaraes-Ferreira L (2014). Role of the phosphocreatine system on energetic homeostasis in skeletal and cardiac muscles. *Einstein* 12(1): 126-31.

[393] Wallimann T, Wyss M, Brdiczka D, Nicolay K, Eppenberger HM. Intracellular compartmentation, structure and function of creatine kinase isoenzymes in tissues with high and fluctuating energy demands: the 'phosphocreatine circuit' for cellular energy homeostasis. Biochem J. 1992;281(Pt 1):21-40. Review.

[394] Wallimann T et al (2011). The creatine kinase system and pleiotropic effects of creatine. *Amino Acids*, 40: 1271-1296.

[395] Wallimann T et al (2011). The creatine kinase system and pleiotropic effects of creatine. *Amino Acids*, 40: 1271-1296.

[396] Wallimann T et al (2011). The creatine kinase system and pleiotropic effects of creatine. *Amino Acids*, 40: 1271-1296.

[397] Wallimann T et al (2011). The creatine kinase system and pleiotropic effects of creatine. *Amino Acids*, 40: 1271-1296.

[398] Kay L, Nicolay K, Wieringa B, Saks V, Wallimann T (2000) Direct evidence for the control of mitochondrial respiration by mitochondrial creatine kinase in oxidative muscle cells in situ. J Biol Chem 275:6937–6944

[399] Wallimann T et al (2011). The creatine kinase system and pleiotropic effects of creatine. *Amino Acids*, 40: 1271-1296.

[400] Bender A, Beckers J, Schneider I, Holter SM, Haack T, Ruthsatz T, Vogt-Weisenhorn DM, Becker L, Genius J, Rujescu D, Irmler M, Mijalski T, Mader M, Quintanilla-Martinez L, Fuchs H, Gailus-Durner V, de Angelis MH, Wurst W, Schmidt J, Klopstock T (2008a) Creatine improves health and survival of mice. Neurobiol Aging 29:1404–1411

[401] Gualano B, Novaes RB, Artioli GG, Freire TO, Coelho DF, Scagliusi FB, Rogeri PS, Roschel H, Ugrinowitsch C, Lancha AH Jr (2008a) Effects of creatine supplementation on glucose tolerance and insulin sensitivity in sedentary healthy males undergoing aerobic training. Amino Acids 34:245–250

[402] Owen L & Sunram-Lea S I (2011). Metabolic Agents that Enhance ATP can Improve Cognitive Functioning: A Review of the Evidence for Glucose, Oxygen, Pyruvate, Creatine, and L-Carnitine. *Nutrients*, 3:735-755.

[403] Rango, M.; Castelli, A.; Scarlato, G. Energetics of 3.5 s neural activation in humans: A 31P MR spectroscopy study. *Magn. Reson. Med.* 1997, *38*, 878–883.

[404] Owen L & Sunram-Lea S I (2011). Metabolic Agents that Enhance ATP can Improve Cognitive Functioning: A Review of the Evidence for Glucose, Oxygen, Pyruvate, Creatine, and L-Carnitine. *Nutrients*, 3:735-755.

[405] Ling, J.; Kritikos, M.; Tiplady, B. Cognitive effects of creatine ethyl ester supplementation. *Behav. Pharmacol.* 2009, *20*, 673–679.

[406] Wallimann T et al (2011). The creatine kinase system and pleiotropic effects of creatine. *Amino Acids*, 40: 1271-1296.

[407] Owen L & Sunram-Lea S I (2011). Metabolic Agents that Enhance ATP can Improve Cognitive Functioning: A Review of the Evidence for Glucose, Oxygen, Pyruvate, Creatine, and L-Carnitine. *Nutrients*, 3:735-755.

[408] Bender A, Samtleben W, Elstner M, Klopstock T (2008b) Long-term creatine supplementation is safe in aged patients with Parkinson disease. Nutr Res 28:172–178

[409] Simopoulous A P (2013). Dietary Omega-3 Fatty Acid Deficiency and High Fructose Intake in the Development of Metabolic Syndrome, Brain Metabolic Abnormalities, and Non-Alcoholic Fatty Liver Disease. *Nutrients*, 5:2901-2923.

[410] Schmitz, G.; Ecker, J. The opposing effects of *n*-3 and *n*-6 fatty acids. *Prog. Lipid Res.* 2008, *47*, 147–155.

[411] Stanhope, K.L.; Schwarz, J.M.; Keim, N.L.; Griffen, S.C.; Bremer, A.A.; Graham, J.L.; Hatcher, B.; Cox, C.L.; Dyachenko, A.; Zhang, W.; *et al.* Consuming fructose-sweetened, not glucose-sweetened, beverages increases visceral adiposity and lipids and decreases insulin sensitivity in overweight/obese humans. *J. Clin. Investig.* 2009, *119*, 1322–1334.

[412] Simopoulous A P (2013). Dietary Omega-3 Fatty Acid Deficiency and High Fructose Intake in the Development of Metabolic Syndrome, Brain Metabolic Abnormalities, and Non-Alcoholic Fatty Liver Disease. *Nutrients*, 5:2901-2923.

[413] Simopoulous A P (2013). Dietary Omega-3 Fatty Acid Deficiency and High Fructose Intake in the Development of Metabolic Syndrome, Brain Metabolic Abnormalities, and Non-Alcoholic Fatty Liver Disease. *Nutrients*, 5:2901-2923.

[414] Simopoulous A P (2013). Dietary Omega-3 Fatty Acid Deficiency and High Fructose Intake in the Development of Metabolic Syndrome, Brain Metabolic Abnormalities, and Non-Alcoholic Fatty Liver Disease. *Nutrients*, 5:2901-2923.

[415] Simopoulous A P (2013). Dietary Omega-3 Fatty Acid Deficiency and High Fructose Intake in the Development of Metabolic Syndrome, Brain Metabolic Abnormalities, and Non-Alcoholic Fatty Liver Disease. *Nutrients*, 5:2901-2923.

[416] Lopez-Huertas, E. The effect of EPA and DHA on metabolic syndrome patients: A systematic review of randomised controlled trials. *Br. J. Nutr.* 2012, *107* (Suppl. 2), 185–194.

[417] Tierney AC et al. Effects of dietary fat modification on insulin sensitivity and on other risk factors of the metabolic syndrome--LIPGENE: a European randomized dietary intervention study. Int J Obes (Lond). 2011 Jun;35(6):800-9.

[418] Kabir, M.; Skurnik, G.; Naour, N.; Pechtner, V.; Meugnier, E.; Rome, S.; Quignard-Boulange, A.; Vidal, H.; Slama, G.; Clement, K.; Guerre-Millo, M.; Rizkalla, S. Treatment for 2 mo with n-3 polyunsaturated fatty acids reduces adiposity and some atherogenic factors but does not improve insulin sensitivity in women with type 2 diabetes: A randomized controlled study. *Am. J. Clin. Nutr.* 2007, *86*, 1670-1679.

[419] British Journal of Nutrition 2002 Oct;88(4):355-63 Eicosapentaenoic and docosapentaenoic acids are the principal products of alpha-linolenic acid metabolism in young men*. Burdge GC, Jones AE, Wootton SA. Institute of Human Nutrition, University of Southampton, Southampton, UK.

[420] Ball D (2015). Metabolic and endocrine response to exercise: sympathoadrenal integration with skeletal muscle. *Journal of Endocrinology*, 224: R79-R95.

[421] Ball D (2015). Metabolic and endocrine response to exercise: sympathoadrenal integration with skeletal muscle. *Journal of Endocrinology*, 224: R79-R95.

[422] Goyaram V, Kohn TA & Ojuka EO 2014 Suppression of the GLUT4 adaptive response to exercise in fructose-fed rats. American Journal of Physiology. Endocrinology and Metabolism 306 E275–E283.

[423] Henderson GC & Alderman BL 2014 Determinants of resting lipid oxidation in response to a prior bout of endurance exercise. Journal of Applied Physiology 116 95–103.

[424] Olesen J, Gliemann L, Biensø R, Schmidt J, Hellsten Y & Pilegaard H 2014 Exercise training, but not resveratrol, improves metabolic and inflammatory status in skeletal muscle of aged men. Journal of Physiology 592 1872–1886.

[425] Pedersen BK 2013 Muscle as a secretory organ. Comprehensive Physiology 3 1337–1362.

[426] Ball D (2015). Metabolic and endocrine response to exercise: sympathoadrenal integration with skeletal muscle. *Journal of Endocrinology*, 224: R79-R95.

[427] Ball D (2015). Metabolic and endocrine response to exercise: sympathoadrenal integration with skeletal muscle. *Journal of Endocrinology*, 224: R79-R95.

[428] Ball D (2015). Metabolic and endocrine response to exercise: sympathoadrenal integration with skeletal muscle. *Journal of Endocrinology*, 224: R79-R95.

[429] Ball D (2015). Metabolic and endocrine response to exercise: sympathoadrenal integration with skeletal muscle. *Journal of Endocrinology*, 224: R79-R95.

[430] Ball D (2015). Metabolic and endocrine response to exercise: sympathoadrenal integration with skeletal muscle. *Journal of Endocrinology*, 224: R79-R95.

[431] Ball D (2015). Metabolic and endocrine response to exercise: sympathoadrenal integration with skeletal muscle. *Journal of Endocrinology*, 224: R79-R95.

[432] Arner P 2005 Human fat cell lipolysis: biochemistry, regulation and clinical role. Best Practice & Research. Clinical Endocrinology & Metabolism 19 471–482.

[433] Howlett K, Galbo H, Lorentsen J, Bergeron R, Zimmerman-Belsing T, Bulow J, Feldt-Rasmussen U & Kjaer M 1999 Effect of adrenaline on
glucose kinetics during exercise in adrenalectomised humans. Journal of Physiology 519 911–921.

[434] Hill, E. ., Zack, E., Battaglini, C., Viru, M., Viru, A. and Hackney, A.C. (2008) Exercise and circulating cortisol levels: The intensity
threshold effect. *Journal of Endocrinological Investigation* **31**, 587-591.

[435] Romijn JA, Coyle EF, Sidossis LS, Gastadelli A, Horowitz JA, Endert E & Wolfe RR 1993 Regulation of endogenous fat and carbohydrate metabolism in relation to exercise intensity and duration. American Journal of Physiology. Endocrinology and Metabolism 265 E380–E391.

[436] Ball D (2015). Metabolic and endocrine response to exercise: sympathoadrenal integration with skeletal muscle. *Journal of Endocrinology*, 224: R79-R95.

[437] Brooks K A & Carter J G (2013). Overtraining, Exercise, and Adrenal Insufficiency. *J Nov Physiother*, 3(125): doi: 10.4172/2165-7025.1000125.

[438] Brooks K A & Carter J G (2013). Overtraining, Exercise, and Adrenal Insufficiency. *J Nov Physiother*, 3(125): doi: 10.4172/2165-7025.1000125.

[439] Brooks K A & Carter J G (2013). Overtraining, Exercise, and Adrenal Insufficiency. *J Nov Physiother*, 3(125): doi: 10.4172/2165-7025.1000125.

[440] Brooks K A & Carter J G (2013). Overtraining, Exercise, and Adrenal Insufficiency. *J Nov Physiother*, 3(125): doi: 10.4172/2165-7025.1000125.

[441] Angeli A, Minetto M, Dovio A, Paccotti P. The overtraining syndrome in athletes: a stress-related disorder. J Endocrinol Invest. 2004; 27:603–612

[442] Baschetti R. Overlap of chronic fatigue syndrome with primary adrenocortical insufficiency. Horm Metab Res. 1999; 31:439.

[443] Brooks K A & Carter J G (2013). Overtraining, Exercise, and Adrenal Insufficiency. *J Nov Physiother*, 3(125): doi: 10.4172/2165-7025.1000125.

[444] S. M. Grundy, B. Hansen, S. C. Smith Jr., J. I. Cleeman, and R. A. Kahn, "American Heart Association; National Heart, Lung, and Blood Institute; American Diabetes Association. Clinical management of metabolic syndrome: report of the American Heart Association/National Heart, Lung, and Blood Institute/American Diabetes Association conference on scientific issues related to management," *Circulation*, vol. 109, no. 4, pp. 551–556, 2004.

[445] The Diabetes Prevention Program Research Group, "The Diabetes Prevention Program (DPP): description of lifestyle intervention," *Diabetes Care*, vol. 25, no. 12, pp. 2165–2171, 2002.

[446] "Clinical Guidelines on the Identification, Evaluation, and Treatment of Overweight and Obesity in Adults. The Evidence Report. National Institutes of Health," *Obesity Research*, vol. 6, supplement 2, pp. 51S–209S, 1998.

[447] Kaur J (2014). A Comprehensive Review on Metabolic Syndrome. *Cardiology Research and Practice*, Article ID 943162.

[448] W. L. Haskell, I.-M. Lee, R. R. Pate et al., "Physical activity and public health: updated recommendation for adults from the American College of Sports Medicine and the American Heart Association," *Circulation*, vol. 116, no. 9, pp. 1081–1093, 2007.

[449] Wierzejska R (2012). Caffeine – common ingredient in a diet and its influence on human health. *Rocz Panstw Zakl Hig*, 63(2): 141-7.

[450] Ibrahim N K & Iftikhar R (2014). Energy drinks: Getting wings but at what health cost? *Pak J Med Sci,* 30(6): 1415-1419.

[451] Lovett R (24 September 2005). "Coffee: The demon drink?". *New Scientist*(2518).

[452] Fredholm BB, Battig K, Holmen J, Nehlig A, Zvartau EE. Actions of caffeine in the brain with special reference to factors that contribute to its widespread use. Pharmacol. Rev. 1999; 51:83

[453] Sepkowitz KA. Energy drinks and caffeine-related adverse effects. JAMA. 2013;309(3):243-244.

[454] Fisone G, Borgkvist A, Usiello A (2004). "Caffeine as a psychomotor stimulant: mechanism of action". *Cell. Mol. Life Sci.* 61 (7–8): 857–72

[455] Burnstock G (2014). Purinergic signalling: from discovery to current developments. *Exp Physiol,* 99(1): 16-34.

[456] Nam H W et al (2012). Adenosine and Glutamate Signaling in Neuron-Glial interactions: Implications in Alcoholism and Sleep Disorders. *Alcohol Clin Exp Res*, 36(7): 1117-1125.

[457] Yegutkin GG (2008). Nucleotide- and nucleoside-converting ectoenzymes: important modulators of purinergic signalling cascade. *Biochim Biophys Acta* 1783, 673–694.

[458] Fredholm B, Chen J-F, Masino SA, Vaugeois J-M. Actions of adeosine at its receptors in the CNS: insights from knckouts and drugs. Annu. Rev. Pharmacol. Toxicol. 2005; 45:385–412.

[459] Chen J-F (2013). Adenosine receptors as drug targets — what are the challenges? *Nat Rev Drug Discov*, 12(4): 265-286.

[460] Chen J-F (2013). Adenosine receptors as drug targets — what are the challenges? *Nat Rev Drug Discov*, 12(4): 265-286.

[461] Elliott MR, et al. Nucleotides released by apoptotic cells act as a find-me signal to promote phagocytic clearance. Nature. 2009; 461:282–286.

[462] Fisone G, Borgkvist A, Usiello A (2004). "Caffeine as a psychomotor stimulant: mechanism of action". *Cell. Mol. Life Sci.* 61 (7–8): 857–72

[463] World of Caffeine (2014). Caffeine and neurotransmitters. http://worldofcaffeine.com/caffeine-and-neurotransmitters/. [Accessed 06/03/15].

[464] Papamichael CM, Aznaouridis KA, Karatzis EN, Karatzi KN, Stamatelopoulos KS, Vamvakou G, et al. Effect of coffee on endothelial function in healthy subjects: the role of caffeine. Clin Sci (Lond). 2005;109(1):55-60.

[465] Mahmud A, Feely J. Acute effect of caffeine on arterial stiffness and aortic pressure waveform. Hypertension. 2001;38(2):227-231.

[466] Usman A, Jawaid A. Hypertension in a young boy: an energy drink effect. BMC Res Notes. 2012;5:591.

[467] Clauson KA, Shields KM, McQueen CE, Persad N. Safety issues associated with commercially available energy drinks. J Am Pharm Assoc. (2003) 2008;48(3):e55-63; quiz e64-7.

[468] Mednick SC, Cai DJ, Kanady J, Drummond SP. Comparing the benefits of caffeine, naps and placebo on verbal, motor and perceptual memory. Behav Brain Res. 2008;193(1):79-86.

[469] Smith A. Effects of caffeine on human behavior. Food Chem Toxicol. 2002;40(9):1243-1255.

[470] Jones SR, Fernyhough C. Caffeine, stress, and proneness to psychosis-like experiences: A preliminary investigation. Personality and Individual Differences. 2009;46(4):562-564.

[471] Sepkowitz KA. Energy drinks and caffeine-related adverse effects. JAMA. 2013;309(3):243-244.

[472] Sepkowitz KA. Energy drinks and caffeine-related adverse effects. JAMA. 2013;309(3):243-244.

[473] Wierzejska R (2012). Caffeine – common ingredient in a diet and its influence on human health. *Rocz Panstw Zakl Hig*, 63(2): 141-7.

[474] Wierzejska R (2012). Caffeine – common ingredient in a diet and its influence on human health. *Rocz Panstw Zakl Hig*, 63(2): 141-7.

[475] Sepkowitz KA. Energy drinks and caffeine-related adverse effects. JAMA. 2013;309(3):243-244.

[476] Ibrahim N K & Iftikhar R (2014). Energy drinks: Getting wings but at what health cost? *Pak J Med Sci,* 30(6): 1415-1419.

[477] Ibrahim N K & Iftikhar R (2014). Energy drinks: Getting wings but at what health cost? *Pak J Med Sci,* 30(6): 1415-1419.

[478] Ibrahim N K & Iftikhar R (2014). Energy drinks: Getting wings but at what health cost? *Pak J Med Sci,* 30(6): 1415-1419.

[479] Sports drinks and energy drinks for children and adolescents: are they appropriate? Pediatrics. 2011;127(6):1182-1189.

[480] Clauson KA, Shields KM, McQueen CE, Persad N. Safety issues associated with commercially available energy drinks. J Am Pharm Assoc. (2003) 2008;48(3):e55-63; quiz e64-7.

[481] Ibrahim N K & Iftikhar R (2014). Energy drinks: Getting wings but at what health cost? *Pak J Med Sci,* 30(6): 1415-1419.

[482] Vos MB, Lavine JE. Dietary fructose in nonalcoholic fatty liver disease. Hepatology. 2013;57(6):2525-2531.

[483] Sepkowitz KA. Energy drinks and caffeine-related adverse effects. JAMA. 2013;309(3):243-244.

[484] Sepkowitz KA. Energy drinks and caffeine-related adverse effects. JAMA. 2013;309(3):243-244.

[485] **Rehm J**, Mathers C, Popova S, Thavorncharoensap M, Teerawattananon Y, Patra J. Global burden of disease and injury and economic cost attributable to alcohol use and alcoholuse disorders. *Lancet* 2009; **373**: 2223-2233

[486] Kim J J et al (2015). Chronic alcohol consumption potentiates the development of diabetes through pancreatic b-cell dysfunction. *World J Biol Chem*, 6(1): 1-5.

[487] Nassar F & Ibdah J A (2014). Role of mitochondria in alcoholic liver disease. *World J Gastroenterol*, 20(9): 2136-2142.

[488] Office of National Statistics (2013). Statistical Bulletin: Adult Drinking Habits in Great Britain, 2013. http://www.ons.gov.uk/ons/dcp171778_395191 [Accesses 06/03/15]

[489] Office of National Statistics (2013). Statistical Bulletin: Adult Drinking Habits in Great Britain, 2013. http://www.ons.gov.uk/ons/dcp171778_395191 [Accesses 06/03/15]

[490] Ferre S & O'Brien M B (2011). Alcohol and Caffeine: The Perfect Storm. *Journal of Caffeine Research*, 1(3): 153-162

[491] Nam H W et al (2012). Adenosine and Glutamate Signaling in Neuron-Glial interactions: Implications in Alcoholism and Sleep Disorders. *Alcohol Clin Exp Res*, 36(7): 1117-1125.

[492] Nam H W et al (2012). Adenosine and Glutamate Signaling in Neuron-Glial interactions: Implications in Alcoholism and Sleep Disorders. *Alcohol Clin Exp Res*, 36(7): 1117-1125.

[493] Ferre S & O'Brien M B (2011). Alcohol and Caffeine: The Perfect Storm. *Journal of Caffeine Research*, 1(3): 153-162

[494] Ferre S & O'Brien M B (2011). Alcohol and Caffeine: The Perfect Storm. *Journal of Caffeine Research*, 1(3): 153-162

[495] HAMS Harm Reduction Network (2012). Alcohol and Dopamine. http://www.hamsnetwork.org/dopamine.pdf. [Accessed 07/03/15].

[496] Ferre S & O'Brien M B (2011). Alcohol and Caffeine: The Perfect Storm. *Journal of Caffeine Research*, 1(3): 153-162.

[497] Miranda-Mendez A, Lugo-Baruqui A, Armendariz-Borunda J. Molecular basis and current treatment for alcoholic liver disease. *Int J Environ Res Public Health* 2010; **7**: 1872-1888/

[498] Méndez-Sánchez N, Almeda-Valdés P, Uribe M. Alcoholic liver disease. An update. *Ann Hepatol* 2005; **4**: 32-42.

[499] Mendenhall CL. Anabolic steroid therapy as an adjunct to diet in alcoholic hepatic steatosis. *Am J Dig Dis* 1968; 13: 783-791.

[500] Deleuran T, Grønbaek H, Vilstrup H, Jepsen P. Cirrhosis and mortality risks of biopsy-verified alcoholic pure steatosis and steatohepatitis: a nationwide registry-based study. *Aliment Pharmacol Ther* 2012; **35**: 1336-1342

[501] Nassar F & Ibdah J A (2014). Role of mitochondria in alcoholic liver disease. *World J Gastroenterol*, 20(9): 2136-2142.

[502] Levitt MD, Li R, DeMaster EG, Elson M, Furne J, Levitt DG. Use of measurements of ethanol absorption from stomach and intestine to assess human ethanol metabolism. *Am J Physiol* 1997; **273**: G951-G957

[503] Schuckit MA. Ethanol and methanol. In: Goodman & Gilman's The Pharmacological Basis of Therapeutics. L.L. Brunton, B.A. Chabner, B.C. Knollmann (Eds). The McGraw-Hill Companies, China 2011; 12e. Available at www.accessmedicine .com/content.aspx?aID = 16666094

[504] Schuckit MA. Ethanol and methanol. In: Goodman & Gilman's The Pharmacological Basis of Therapeutics. L.L. Brunton, B.A. Chabner, B.C. Knollmann (Eds). The McGraw-Hill Companies, China 2011; 12e. Available at www.accessmedicine .com/content.aspx?aID = 16666094

[505] Nassar F & Ibdah J A (2014). Role of mitochondria in alcoholic liver disease. *World J Gastroenterol*, 20(9): 2136-2142.

[506] Schuckit MA. Ethanol and methanol. In: Goodman & Gilman's The Pharmacological Basis of Therapeutics. L.L. Brunton, B.A. Chabner, B.C. Knollmann (Eds). The McGraw-Hill Companies, China 2011; 12e. Available at www.accessmedicine .com/content.aspx?aID = 16666094

[507] Schuckit MA. Ethanol and methanol. In: Goodman & Gilman's The Pharmacological Basis of Therapeutics. L.L. Brunton, B.A. Chabner, B.C. Knollmann (Eds). The McGraw-Hill Companies, China 2011; 12e. Available at www.accessmedicine .com/content.aspx?aID = 16666094

[508] Nassar F & Ibdah J A (2014). Role of mitochondria in alcoholic liver disease. *World J Gastroenterol*, 20(9): 2136-2142.

[509] Gordon ER. Alcohol-induced mitochondrial changes in the liver. *Recent Dev Alcohol* 1984; **2**: 143-158.

[510] Nassar F & Ibdah J A (2014). Role of mitochondria in alcoholic liver disease. *World J Gastroenterol*, 20(9): 2136-2142.

[511] Nassar F & Ibdah J A (2014). Role of mitochondria in alcoholic liver disease. *World J Gastroenterol*, 20(9): 2136-2142.

[512] Nassar F & Ibdah J A (2014). Role of mitochondria in alcoholic liver disease. *World J Gastroenterol*, 20(9): 2136-2142.

[513] Parlesak A, Schäfer C, Schütz T, Bode JC, Bode C. Increased intestinal permeability to macromolecules and endotoxemia in patients with chronic alcohol abuse in different stages of alcohol-induced liver disease. *J Hepatol* 2000; **32**: 742-747

[514] Voight R M et al (2013). Circadian Disruption: Potential implications in inflammatory and Metabolic diseases Associated With Alcohol. *Alcohol Research,* 35(1): 87-96.

[515] Voight R M et al (2013). Circadian Disruption: Potential implications in inflammatory and Metabolic diseases Associated With Alcohol. *Alcohol Research,* 35(1): 87-96.

[516] 22217099Coogan, a.n., andWYse, C.a.neuroimmunology of thecircadian clock. *Brain Research*1232:104–112, 2008.

[517] Dimitrov S.; lange, T.; FehM, h.l.; andBorn, J.a regulato-ry role of prolactin, growth hormone, and corticosteroidsfor human T-cell production of cytokines. *Brain,Behavior, and Immunity*18:368–374, 2004

[518] Voight R M et al (2013). Circadian Disruption: Potential implications in inflammatory and Metabolic diseases Associated With Alcohol. *Alcohol Research,* 35(1): 87-96.

[519] Voight R M et al (2013). Circadian Disruption: Potential implications in inflammatory and Metabolic diseases Associated With Alcohol. *Alcohol Research,* 35(1): 87-96.

Printed in Great Britain
by Amazon